Advanced Praise for

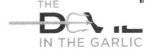

IN THE GARLIC

"Sulfur, and its metabolism, are in the category of most important but least well understood areas in all of medicine. Often relegated to a simplistic corner of biochemistry, sulfur metabolism is intricate and widly impactful on human health. In addition its import in oncology care cannot be overstated. In this seminal work Dr. Nigh lays out the metabolism and chemistry of this important system and its relationship to health and disease. This is a must-read for any health care provider."

—DR. PAUL S. ANDERSON, *co-author, Outside the Box Cancer Therapies*

"Dr. Nigh is a brilliant, experienced physician with a wealth of knowledge on this underappreciated topic. Understanding sulfur is extremely important for health and particularly for complex mysterious illness."

—ALLISON SIEBECKER, ND

"Dr. Greg Nigh is an original thinker of the highest caliber. I pay attention to anything he writes. Here is an example of why that is. In this book he presents us with a new theory of illness, a new idea that explains certain chronic disease issues, and gives us the solutions. As I read this, several patients came to mind, those who did not respond well to what I thought should have improved their health. Now, I have a new understanding of these problem patients. He explained so much in here, from how to interpret genetic markers to the impact of glyphosate, all tied around sulfur metabolism. This book is a refresher course in current medicine along with Greg's advances in thinking. It is a gem."

—JARED ZEFF, ND, LAc

"In reading this book, you will learn a lot about biology and chemistry and water's special properties. You will come to appreciate how fascinating biochemistry can be, but also, perhaps more importantly, you will learn how to change your lifestyle in ways that will promote long-lasting good health."

—STEPHANIE SENEFF, Senior Research Scientist, MIT

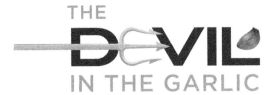

THE DEVIL
IN THE GARLIC

THE

D&VIL

IN THE GARLIC

HOW SULFUR IN YOUR FOOD

CAN CAUSE ANXIETY, HOT FLASHES, IBS, BRAIN FOG,

MIGRAINES, SKIN PROBLEMS, AND MORE, AND

A PROGRAM TO HELP YOU *FEEL GREAT AGAIN*

Greg Nigh, ND, LAc

Author to please complete or confirm text in red below. Website links
included for your convenience to purchase your ISBNs, and to research
Library of Congress and PCIP Data Block information.

Copyrighted Material

The Devil in the Garlic: How Sulfur in Your Food Can Cause
Anxiety, Hot Flashes, IBS, Brain Fog, Migraines, Skin Problems,
and More, and a Program to Help You Feel Great Again

Copyright © 2020 by Greg Nigh. All Rights Reserved.

All rights reserved. Published by Wellness Ink Publishing. No part of this pub-
lication may be reproduced, stored in or introduced into any retrieval system,
or transmitted in any form, or by any means, including photocopying, record-
ing or other electronic or mechanical methods, without the prior written per-
mission of the author, except in the case of brief quotations embodied in critical
reviews and certain other noncommercial uses permitted by copyright law.

For information about this title or to order other books and/
or electronic media, contact the publisher:

Wellness Ink Publishing
Montreal, Quebec, Canada
http://immersionhealthpdx.com
drnigh@immersionhealthpdx.com

Library of Congress Control Number: 2020903974

ISBNs
Softcover: 978-1-988645-33-9
eBook: 978-1-988645-34-6
Audio: 978-1-988645-35-3

Printed in the United States of America

Cover and Interior design: 1106 Design

Disclaimer

A Note to Readers

This book is for informational purposes only and is not intended as a substitute for the advice and care of your health provider. As with all health advice, please consult with a qualified health provider to make sure this program is appropriate for your individual circumstances. The author and publisher expressly disclaim responsibility for any adverse effects that may result from the application, use or misuse of the information contained in this book.

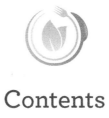

Contents

Contents

Foreword

T his book is a delightful read for anyone who is fascinated by chemistry and an essential read for anyone who suffers from sulfur sensitivity problems. Dr. Nigh has a special talent for describing complicated metabolic pathways in terms that are both entertaining and comprehensible to the lay public. He is very knowledgeable on his subject matter, since many of the patients he treats suffer from sulfur sensitivity issues. He reveals the magic properties of water in colorful terms, and he shows how derangements in sulfur homeostasis can lead to a wide range of diseases, including small intestinal bacterial overgrowth (SIBO), inflammatory bowel disease, fatigue, skin conditions, menopausal symptoms and food allergies.

I have come to believe that systemic sulfate deficiency is a key driver behind many modern diseases. Furthermore, I believe that glyphosate, the active ingredient in the pervasive herbicide Roundup, is the main cause of this sulfate deficiency problem. Critically, Roundup can cause a person's digestive system to become unwelcoming to sulfur-containing foods such as garlic, which eventually leads to a severe sulfur deficiency problem as they naturally avoid these foods.

Dr. Nigh also explains how glyphosate can disrupt sulfur handling by the body, and he offers good advice for how to heal your body if you are dealing with difficult health issues brought on by imbalances in the gut microbiome, and derailments in enzymes like sulfite oxidase (SuOx), PAPS synthase (PAPSS) and cystathionine beta synthase (CBS). These enzymes play essential roles in maintaining proper balance among the various biologically active sulfur-containing molecules. In reading this book, you will learn a lot about biology and chemistry and water's special properties. You will come to appreciate how fascinating biochemistry can be, but also, perhaps more importantly, you will learn how to change your lifestyle in ways that will promote long-lasting good health.

—Stephanie Seneff
Senior Research Scientist, MIT

Acknowledgments

There are a few people who have contributed enormously to this book and the ideas it contains. First and foremost I want to thank Maria Palmer, the nutrition therapist I have worked in collaboration with clinically for over a decade and whose culinary genius has consistently turned my various ideas into delicious new recipes and practical dietary programs for our patients. I'm also grateful to Stephanie Seneff for introducing me to the topic of sulfur and its metabolic importance, and for her ongoing willingness to share ideas and research that I can then mine for clinical applications. The text itself has been made dramatically more readable through the work of my editor Helen Wilkie, and Lynda Goldman's expert guidance on lining up the resources to turn a manuscript into a book has made the process remarkably painless. Finally, I want to thank my parents for their relentless support and many years encouraging me to start writing books. I take full credit for any errors or inconsistencies.

Introduction

"If sulfur metabolism is such a big deal with respect to health and illness, why have I never heard of this problem?"

That's a very good question, and one that continues to mystify me. I stumbled onto this topic almost by accident, and it was only a string of lucky coincidences that ultimately led to the set of therapies you will read about in this book. In order to give some context for the protocol I'll be describing, I'll briefly relate how sulfur issues came to my attention in the first place.

Early in my career as a naturopathic physician, which began in February 2002, I started utilizing an elimination diet with most of my patients. I found it to be the single most beneficial therapy I could prescribe, and I was amazed by the wide range of chronic symptoms that diminish, or even completely resolve, once reactive foods were eliminated from the diet. However, an elimination diet can't eliminate everything, and working with hundreds of patients over time I noticed patterns common among those who seemed not to respond well to the standard elimination diet.

By early 2012 I had started paying attention to symptoms that seemed to be correlated to high intake of foods containing sulphur. These foods were not specifically eliminated during the elimination diet, and in fact often people would eat *more* of these foods since other foods were restricted by the diet. I noticed, too, that specific sulfur-related blood tests for these same people seemed peculiar to me (details on that later). I was already working in collaboration with a nutrition therapist, and she put together an initial set of low-sulfur guidelines for us to utilize with appropriate patients. Even in those early stages we saw some startling changes in symptoms taking place.

In late 2012 I read an article related to the role of sulfate in the body, written by Dr. Stephanie Seneff of MIT. After some brief email exchanges, we arranged a phone conversation so that I could get some follow-up questions answered. It so happened that the nutrition therapist I was working with, Maria Palmer, was in the room during that conversation and was able to hear half of what was discussed. Maria is a Certified GAPS Practitioner who was implementing the GAPS diet with some patients, in addition to several other therapeutic diets I might suggest. GAPS, or Gut and Psychology Syndrome, is a therapeutic diet commonly utilized in the treatment of depression, anxiety, and a range of other mental/emotional symptoms.

Dr. Seneff and I discussed the ways in which disrupted sulfate production and metabolism might lead to various health-related issues. Maria, hearing my half of this conversation, started connecting some dots that had troubled her with some of her GAPS patients. While many had dramatic improvements on the GAPS diet, there were several who seemed to struggle with symptoms that were assumed to be "detox" symptoms: brain fog, fatigue, rashes, digestive upset, and more. She realized at that point that the GAPS diet is very heavily loaded with foods containing sulfur. Maybe those patients having symptoms weren't actually detoxing; maybe they were having trouble metabolizing all that sulfur.

The next piece of the puzzle that fell into place for me had to do with the pioneering research of Gerald Pollack, PhD, a researcher in the College of Engineering at the University of Washington. He brought to light the way that water forms a unique structure when it encounters surfaces with a negative charge. I found this information shocking because our bodies are filled with negatively charged surfaces. As I learned from Dr. Seneff, the negative charge is supplied by none other than sulfur! Putting it all together, it became clear how disrupted sulfur metabolism led to a loss of water structure in the body, which led to a wide range of symptoms and diseases.

Over time, Maria revised and updated the low-sulfur diet protocol, and I dove more deeply into researching nutrients, metabolic pathways, related genetic polymorphisms, and supporting therapies that might augment the dietary protocol. We have each continued to expand our knowledge around this topic and modify the protocol accordingly. This book is, in many ways, the clinical application of the ideas that Dr. Seneff and a few others have put together about sulfur metabolism and its relationship to disease.

The overarching goal of this protocol is to reduce the inflow of dietary sulfur while maximizing the outflow of the symptom-producing sulfur metabolites, hydrogen sulfide and sulfite. At the same time, it is critical that the body have access to adequate amounts of sulfate. It may sound confusing now, but in the chapters that follow you will hear so much about these compounds that it will be abundantly clear how each is contributing to health and to disease.

There is no such thing as a general protocol that will work right for everyone. Over the course of implementation I commonly adjust nutrients, and Maria adjusts the dietary component—not always, but often. That said, there are some elements of the protocol that apply to almost everyone in almost every situation, and the large majority of patients who have sulfur metabolism issues will receive substantial symptom relief by implementing the basics presented in this book.

My intention is not to suggest that sulfur metabolism issues can explain *all* symptoms. There are many reasons someone might experience night sweats, for example, or dermatitis, or anxiety, or indigestion, or many other symptoms. The important point is that these symptoms could be related to sulfur metabolism issues. If they are, then it's a good thing to figure that out.

The purpose of this book is to help you do that.

The chapters will progress from an overview of sulfur metabolism, through how it becomes impaired, and finally to the therapies for getting it working again. Along the way a few topics will be encountered more than once, each time going a bit deeper into its role in the big picture of sulfur. Sulfur metabolism is a complicated topic and the science will deepen as we progress, especially through the first four chapters, but I will keep it all as clear as possible. Some might prefer to skip those details. By the end you will have a more advanced understanding of sulfur metabolism than the vast majority of physicians, and you'll have the knowledge you need to get it working again.

1

Overview of Sulfur

It seems like it doesn't make sense.

Some of the healthiest foods—the ones we are commonly told to eat in abundance—contain fairly high amounts of sulfur. These include the cruciferous vegetables such as broccoli and cauliflower, the alliums such as garlic and onion, and many other "healthy" foods.

The fact is, they *are* healthy, so long as you don't have a problem metabolizing the sulfur they contain. In this book I'm going to explain to you how to tell if sulfur might be contributing to any of a wide range of symptoms you might experience. These symptoms could be sporadic and short-lived, or they could be symptoms you have struggled with for years, or even decades. I've seen them all be dramatically reduced and even disappear completely in the span of just a week or two through the use of the assessment and treatment program I'll describe in this book.

But first, it is important to understand why you need dietary sulfur in the first place, and then how sulfur might have come to be a problem for you. After all, it is true that our bodies need a constant supply of sulfur in order to maintain our overall health and the integrity of our cells and tissues. The more you understand about what sulfur is trying to do in your body, the better you'll understand the rationale behind the therapies that help to "unlock" sulfur metabolism.

What's the Big Deal about Sulfur?

Sulfur is the third most abundant mineral element in the body, behind calcium and phosphorus,[1] with the average-size adult body containing around 130 grams of sulfur. Compare this to iron, a mineral that most of us are much more familiar with. The average adult female has a total of about 3.5 grams of iron in her body, and the average male has about 4 grams. Yet in spite of sulfur's abundance in the body and its central involvement in virtually every vital function, very few doctors have a broad understanding of the roles that sulfur plays in health and disease.

The only relevant source of sulfur for our bodies is dietary, either in the food we eat or in the water we drink. In fact, those who get their drinking water from a well often have quite high levels of sulfur compounds in their water, especially inorganic sulfate, SO_4.[2] The incoming sulfur has to be processed before it is put to use in a number of ways.

Before I go any further, I need to explain a little bit about what I mean when I refer to sulfur in the body and its processing. Sulfur comes into the body in several different forms, meaning that a sulfur atom (or two or many) can be bound to some other atoms that are contained in our food or drink. Sulfur might be bound to oxygen, such as in sulfur dioxide (SO_2), sulfite (SO_3), or sulfate (SO_4). Sulfur might be bound to carbon as it is in proteins, in which case it is called a "thiol." It can also be bound to other sulfur atoms within larger molecules, as it is in garlic and onions, in which case that molecule is called a "disulfide."

Cast of Characters			
Sulfur (S)	**Sulfite (SO3)**	**Hydrogen sulfide (H2S)**	**Sulfate (SO4)**
😐	😩 😫	😟 🙂	😁

---

1 M.E. Nimni, B. Han, F. Cordoba, "Are we getting enough sulfur in our diet?" *Nutrition & Metabolism.* 2007;4:24. doi:10.1186/1743-7075-4-24.

2 Paul F. Hudak, "Sulfate and chloride concentrations in Texas aquifers." *Environment International* 26.1–2 (2000): 55–61.

Whatever form the sulfur takes, a large portion of it needs to be converted to SO_4. This process happens through the action of several enzymes, and I'm going to be talking about most of these enzymes more in later chapters. For now, the important point is that SO_4 in particular is a primary end product of dietary sulfur. Without adequate SO_4 around, a lot of things start to fall apart. To help understand what some of those problems are, you need to know more about some of the essential roles for sulfur and SO_4 in the body. I will be covering these in much more detail later, but I want to give you an initial orientation before getting further into the details.

Protein

Proteins are made up of building blocks called amino acids. There are 20 different amino acids that can build proteins, two of the most abundant being cysteine and methionine. The reason these two are important is that they both contain sulfur, as you can see from the "S" in the diagrams below. I will have more to say about cysteine and methionine in later chapters.

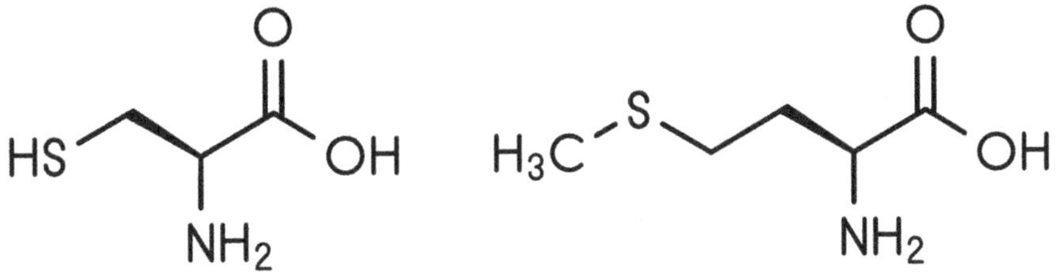

Figure 1. *cysteine*   *methionine*

For now it is important to know that you can't build muscles, produce hormones, or carry out any number of other important functions in your body without adequate amounts of these two amino acids to build the proteins that carry them out.

3

Connective Tissue

The two most familiar forms of connective tissue are those that are commonly injured or torn: ligaments and tendons. In fact, there are other types of connective tissue in the body. Connective tissue is the "stuff" that fills the spaces between our cells. It is what blood vessels, skin, and the white part of your eyes (the sclera) are made of. While connective tissue can play a wide variety of roles depending on where it is, it all contains large amounts of sulfur, more specifically SO_4. Without adequate amounts of SO_4 the connective tissue loses its integrity, leading to ruptures, tears, and other problems.

Detoxification

Sulfur is a central element in our body's ability to protect itself

---

Blood: The Unexpected Connective Tissue

It is easy to see why ligaments and tendons are considered connective tissue, but blood?

Consider this: Connective tissue connects, it spans the distance between cells, between bones, and fills just about any other space that needs to be filled. In that sense, blood fits the bill. Blood is a three-dimensional matrix spanning literally thousands of miles within the body, connecting the cells, tissues, and organs.

---

against the various toxic substances we come into contact with regularly as we move through the modern world.[3] Medications, solvents and other chemicals, heavy metals—these and other compounds are rendered much less harmful in the body through a process happening in the liver called "sulfation." As you might guess, this involves sticking an SO_4 molecule onto a toxic substance to make it less toxic.

---

3 M.W.H. Coughtrie (2002). "Sulfation through the looking glass—recent advances in sulfotransferase research for the curious." *The Pharmacogenomics Journal*, 2(5), 297.

Antioxidant

Antioxidants do just what their name suggests: They help fight against the harmful activities of substances called oxidants. Most people are familiar with antioxidant vitamins such as C, E, and A. Other common antioxidants include lipoic acid, glutathione, and MSM. These last three, as well as several other important antioxidants, owe much of their beneficial effect to the presence of sulfur in their molecular structure. When these sulfur compounds bump into harmful oxidants in cells and tissue, sulfur can render them far less damaging to the body.

Immune Function

Anytime the body needs to fight an infection, the demand for sulfur rises dramatically.[4] The same is also true of inflammation. Both acute and chronic infections require a steady supply of sulfur in order to build the various molecules needed to fight the infection. Likewise, both acute and chronic inflammation typically lead to the breakdown of tissue that has to be rebuilt, and rebuilding new tissue will almost certainly require plenty of sulfur.

Hormone and Neurotransmitter Metabolism

A large number of hormones and neurotransmitters move around in your body with a SO_4 molecule attached to them. These include estrogen, testosterone, progesterone, DHEA, melatonin, dopamine, serotonin, thyroid hormones, and many others. The activity of these substances can change dramatically based upon the presence or absence of the sulfate.

This is a short list of the very large number of roles that sulfur in its various forms plays in the body. It helps to illustrate why it is so important that we maintain an adequate supply, and it also hints at some of the problems that can arise when sulfur cannot be adequately utilized

---

4 R. Grimble, "Sulfur amino acids, gluthathione, and immune function." Glutathione and Sulfur Amino Acids in Human Health and Disease, edited by Roberta M, Guiseppe M. Hoboken, NJ: John Wiley and Sons, Inc. (2009), 273-288.

in the body. There are a few more very important roles for sulfate in the body, but I'll put those off until the next chapter because it will make more sense with a bit of background first.

Chapter 1 has offered a very brief overview of the vital roles that sulfur in general, and sulfate in particular, play in normal body function and health maintenance. In Chapter 2 I'll go into much more detail about how sulfur enters and is transformed in the body, ultimately supplying us with much-needed sulfate.

2

Understanding Pathways and Functions

Now that you understand the critical roles sulfur plays in the body, it's time to dig more deeply into the enzymes, nutrients, and pathways that are involved in proper sulfur metabolism. We will even discuss some genes that can have an impact on how this all works. Don't worry, this is not going to be filled with technical details, but it is going to set the stage for what's to follow in Chapter 3: how it can all go wrong. I will be talking in more detail about genes and nutrients in later chapters, but we will touch on those topics here.

Most processes that happen in the body are dizzyingly complex and complicated. That said, below are a few images that leave out hundreds of details while conveying some of the most important points about what happens to sulfur once it is consumed in the diet.

I realize this diagram looks like a bit of a mess, but it will become clear as I refer to it often, picking it apart as we come to understand the big picture of sulfur and how it moves through the body.

Each arrow indicates an important pathway. Even the H_2S and SO_3 that are produced are important components of a well-working sulfur cycle in the body. But if any of these pathways runs too fast or too slow— or more commonly it's some combination of the two—then problems *and symptoms* start to develop. Let's work our way down the path from dietary sulfur to inorganic sulfate.

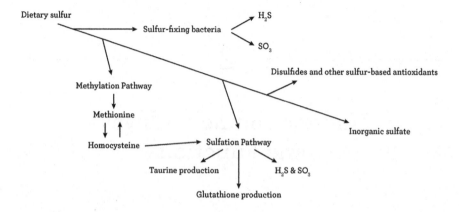

Figure 2. *Fate of Dietary Sulfur*

Methylation Pathway

Methylation has garnered a lot of headlines, many tens of thousands of blog posts, and endless forum discussions, so much so that it has now become an industry unto itself. We do not have space to go into the details of methylation in this book, but since that pathway is intimately tied to the sulfation pathway, a look at its most important aspects is in order.

The methylation pathway is all about generating small molecules called methyl groups, written as CH_3. Methyl groups get attached to an enormous number of other molecules in order to alter their activity in the body. These methyl groups become attached to DNA to regulate gene expression, attached to hormones and neurotransmitters to facilitate their breakdown, shuffled among immune cells to activate and/or inactivate as needed, and so much more.

The methylation cycle "spins" by converting dietary methionine, through a series of reactions, into homocysteine. Each time that conversion happens, a methyl group is created. In order to keep the cycle going, homocysteine needs to be converted back into methionine, and here is where the connection to the sulfur pathway is most apparent. Both methionine and homocysteine are sulfur-containing amino acids. If the conversion of homocysteine back "up" to methionine is slowed down for any reason, that can cause an excess of homocysteine to build up. Whether built up or not, if conditions are right the homocysteine can be drawn "down" the sulfation pathway. So, to start with, let's review some things that can slow the methylation cycle.

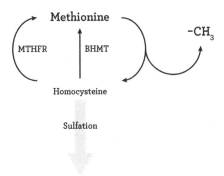

Figure 3. Methylation cycle

Required Nutrients

A very large percentage of chemical reactions that happen in the body happen by way of enzymes. Enzymes are proteins that facilitate a chemical reaction between other molecules, and in order to function optimally they will very commonly have vitamin and/or mineral "cofactors." Deficiencies of these cofactors can lead to slow enzyme activity, and overt lack of cofactors can bring some enzyme activity to a complete halt. The methylation cycle involves several necessary cofactors. A few of the key nutrients are the following:

1. Vitamin B12 (cobalamin)—A methylated form of this vitamin, called methylcobalamin, donates the methyl group to homocysteine, converting it back to methionine.

2. Methylfolate (also known as 5-methyltetrahydrofolate, or 5-MTHF)—This is the active form of folic acid. Once B12 has donated its methyl group to homocysteine, methylfolate has to re-methylate the B12 so it can do it all over again.

Andrea's Ulcerative Colitis

Andrea was the spouse of a patient who had been coming to the clinic and who had experienced significant improvement with his condition. He convinced Andrea to come in. Her story was both typical and heartbreaking.

She had suffered from significant digestive symptoms for as long as she could remember. As a young and vital kid she just dealt with it, assuming it was how people feel when they eat. She grew up in a small town in the Midwest where her uncle owned a pizza parlor. Andrea spent many summers and countless hours helping out in the shop, and of course eating the delicious pizza and other Italian food served up daily.

When she left the Midwest, she took her taste for Italian food with her. Dining out would tend toward Italian restaurants, and meals cooked at home were typically heavy with garlic, onions, shallots, capers, and other staples of Italian cuisine. Unfortunately, she also brought her digestive symptoms along with her as well, and as she got older the symptoms continued to worsen.

Her gut was bad. She had fairly constant abdominal pain, with intermittent cramping. She would occasionally have blood or mucus in her stools, and she alternated between diarrhea and constipation. She said there was virtually never a time when she didn't have some degree of discomfort in her gut.

But her gut was only part of her problems. Andrea was now married with two young children, and her fatigue was so profound that she felt unable to engage in normal family life and activities. She spent long hours lying around, and napping during the day was a necessity. When she was up and around, she constantly struggled with brain fog. She found it difficult to remember what she had been told even within a few minutes of being told. She could no longer maintain her attention long enough to read, something she once considered a favorite pastime.

By this point she had tried several different strategies with her diet, attempting to find out if anything she was eating was triggering her symptoms. While she would receive modest relief with some types of dietary elimination, it was always temporary. The same was true of various supplements she tried. Nothing gave her more than slight improvements.

Andrea had seen enough doctors by this point that she wasn't excited to be seeing another one. However, within just a few minutes of gathering her history, the most likely cause of her problems was apparent to me: She was not metabolizing sulfur appropriately. The byproducts of sulfur metabolism could explain every one of Andrea's symptoms. Working in conjunction with the nutrition therapist in my office, I had Andrea go through the protocol described in this book.

Within just one week Andrea reported that every one of her symptoms had dramatically improved. It was the first time she could recall having no abdominal discomfort, no brain fog, and good energy throughout her days. She was engaged in her parenting, cooking meals for the family—with modified recipes, of course—and mostly in disbelief that such relatively small changes to her diet and supplements could produce such significant change in her well-being.

3. Vitamin B2 (riboflavin)—This vitamin supports the activity of one of the most important enzymes in the methylation cycle, commonly referred to by its abbreviation MTHF, which is made by the somewhat infamous gene called MTHFR.

4. Magnesium—This is the most common mineral cofactor among the reactions of methylation.

If any of these or other important cofactors are missing, the methylation cycle slows, homocysteine can build up, and more homocysteine can move down the sulfur pathway than it would under optimal nutrient conditions.

Methylation Genes

Remember, genes make proteins, and many of those proteins function as enzymes. Enzymes are a particular kind of protein that will make a chemical reaction happen quickly where, without the enzyme, it would happen slowly or not at all.

Again, whole books have been written on the topic of genes related to the methylation cycle. I'm only going to mention a handful that have the most direct impact on the efficiency of that cycle, and thus on keeping homocysteine moving and not building up.

1. MTHFR, or methylenetetrahydrofolate reductase, if you want to impress your friends—This is one of the most studied genes in all of medicine, and for good reason. The enzyme encoded by this gene keeps folate methylated, which keeps B12 methylated, which keeps homocysteine methylated. There are some well-established polymorphisms (see sidebar, next page) in this gene that can have a big impact on how efficiently it operates. A primary function of this gene is to keep the body supplied with active folate, so supplementation can be appropriate for those

with reduced gene activity. Polymorphisms in this gene cause the enzyme it codes for to slow down, which can be a significant issue.

2. BHMT, or betaine-homo-cysteine-N-methyltrans-ferase—Homocysteine has two routes back to methionine within the methylation cycle. One route depends on MTHFR, and the other on BHMT. Polymorphisms can slow down the cycle here too, increasing the pool of homocysteine that can exit through the sulfation pathway. A nutrient in the B vitamin family called choline speeds up the function of this enzyme.

3. MTR, or 5-methyltetra-hydrofolate-homocysteine methyltransferase—The enzyme made by this gene facilitates the actual transfer of a methyl group from vitamin B12 to homocysteine, thereby converting homocysteine back to methionine.

Primer on Genes

Think of genes as made of beads on a string. The beads are called "nucleotides," and a given gene might have anywhere from less than 100 to several thousand of these beads lined up. There are four different types of beads, and there is a "typical" way these four beads line up on in any given gene.

If a single one of those beads is replaced by a different bead that is not as typical in that location, it is called a "Single Nucleotide Polymorphism," or "snip." Snips can range from being completely harmless, to causing serious illness.

Many snips are now known to have a mild-to-moderate impact on the enzyme coded by that gene. Knowing what those snipped enzymes do and what nutrients they need to work optimally is the main point of a thorough genetic review.

Many B vitamins, including B6, B12, and folate, will speed up the activity of this enzyme. There are polymorphisms in this gene that will, again, significantly alter the activity of the enzyme it codes for, resulting in impaired recycling of vitamin B12.

4. MTRR, or (just when you thought these names couldn't get any longer) 5-methyltetrahydrofolate-homocysteine methyltransferase reductase—The enzyme coded by this gene restores the MTR enzyme so that *it* can keep doing its job. You see how these are all interlinked. When one doesn't work correctly, it ricochets through the system to mess it all up. The same B vitamins for MTR will work on this one as well.

Sulfation Pathway

Sulfation is a general term for the various pathways sulfur moves through in order to be incorporated into some important molecules. Like methylation, sulfation is critical for life. Four extremely important molecules are generated via these sulfation pathways.

1. Glutathione—This is one of the most important antioxidant and detoxifying molecules in the body. Glutathione is responsible for binding and eliminating heavy metals, reducing inflammation, quenching free radicals before they cause damage,

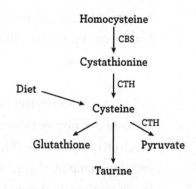

Figure 4. Sulfation Pathways

protecting nerves and the brain from toxic chemicals, and much more. Our bodies need a constant supply of glutathione. Since cysteine, one of the amino acids that contain sulfur, is part of the glutathione molecule, the sulfation pathway is required to generate it.

2. Taurine—This is an interesting molecule, a sulfur-containing amino acid that is not used to build proteins. Instead, taurine is an important component of bile acids, thereby assisting with fat digestion and maintaining the health of the gallbladder. It is also a key nutrient for heart function and cardiovascular health. Taurine can also help with stress by activating the "rest and digest" parasympathetic branch of the nervous system. We get some taurine in our diet, but we also continuously make taurine via sulfation.

3. Cysteine—As mentioned before, cysteine is an amino acid containing sulfur. In fact, cysteine accounts for the majority of dietary sulfur for those who are not vegetarian. Much of the dietary cysteine is utilized via the sulfation pathway. At the same time, our bodies are able to make cysteine via those same sulfation pathways.

4. Pyruvate—Pyruvate doesn't contain sulfur in its structure, but it is a vital by-product of the sulfation pathway. Pyruvate is used in the body predominantly for energy production.

Some Required Nutrients

I'll be going into specific nutrient deficiencies that impact the sulfation pathway in more detail later. For now, three key nutrients are worth mentioning:

1. Vitamin B6 (pyridoxine)—This vitamin is a cofactor for many of the chemical reactions that take place along the sulfation pathway. Either too much or too little of it can cause problems.

2. Iron—Iron is necessary for building sulfite oxidase (SUOX), one of the key enzymes in sulfation. This enzyme is necessary for converting SO_3 to SO_4. We are going to be talking much more about sulfite oxidase in later chapters. Since iron is necessary for its production, and since iron deficiency is not an uncommon problem, you can already see where sulfur metabolism starts to overlap with some other health issues.

3. Molybdenum (abbreviated as Mo)—This funky-sounding mineral is put to only a few uses in the body, but they are very significant uses. In the processing of sulfur, Mo is a cofactor for that same SUOX enzyme that iron is needed to build. We only need very small amounts of Mo in our diet to supply the need, but eating an insufficient amount or increasing the demand for the Mo-dependent enzymes can cause problems.

Sulfation Genes

As with methylation, the enzymes needed to carry out sulfation are built by a few key genes. Here, too, polymorphisms can lead to issues, either pushing too much or not enough sulfur down the sulfation pathway. These are the main players. We will discuss more genes later once we get into the nitty-gritty.

1. CBS (cystathionine beta synthase)—This gene builds the enzyme that acts as the "gatekeeper" at the beginning of the sulfation pathway. CBS links the methylation cycle to sulfation by processing homocysteine "down" toward sulfation. It is easy to see why speeding this enzyme up or slowing it down would both have a large impact on how much homocysteine moves through sulfation. This enzyme is dependent upon the active form of vitamin B6, known as pyridoxal-5-phosphate (P5P). Taking excessive amounts of this nutrient can inadvertently lead to

---

Sulfites and Alcohol
Molybdenum at the Crossroads

In addition to SUOX activity, molybdenum is needed for another important enzyme to do its job. Called aldehyde dehydrogenase (ALDH), this is the enzyme that breaks down the substance that causes hangovers from drinking excessively, called acetaldehyde.

If Mo is in short supply, it results in sulfites hanging out in the body, and it also results in a potentially exaggerated response to drinking even small amounts of alcohol. For this reason I always ask those I suspect of having a sulfur issue how they feel if they drink alcohol. Most will say that they can only have a very small amount and only occasionally because it makes them feel terrible otherwise. It is also common for people to respond that they can't drink at all anymore due to the severity of their reaction to it.

A response like this not only helps to confirm that there is a sulfur metabolism issue, but also that a lack of or inability to utilize Mo might be one of the causes.

---

overstimulation of the CBS enzyme. It is important to know that two by-products of this enzyme's activity are H_2S and SO_3. We will be discussing those in much greater detail later.

2. CTH (cystathionine gamma lyase, also abbreviated as CSE)— Like CBS, the enzyme coded by this gene shows up in multiple places in sulfation pathways. Polymorphisms alter the speed of the enzyme, and like CBS, it is also dependent upon P5P.

3. SUOX (sulfite oxidase)—The proper function of this gene is crucial for sulfur metabolism. In this gene, too, there are polymorphisms that can dramatically impact the function of the encoded enzyme. It is essential to take both nutrients and polymorphisms into account when assessing the role this gene and its related enzyme might be playing in symptoms. This will be discussed in more detail in Chapter 3.

Again, I will have much more to say about these sulfation pathways and related genes in later chapters. For now it will help to have an overview of the key players.

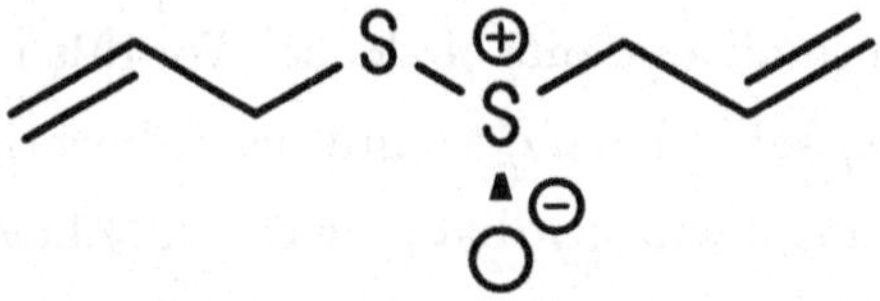

Figure 5. Disulfide bond

Disulfides and Sulfur-Based Antioxidants

Many sulfur-containing foods, such as garlic and broccoli, are known to be healthy and loaded with antioxidants. In fact many of those health-promoting properties are due to disulfides. For example, allicins are a group of sulfur compounds produced by garlic once the cells have been damaged by bacteria, molds, or mechanical insult (crushing it or chewing it up, for example). The image above shows the prominent position of the two sulfurs bonded together within allicin compounds.

Often these disulfide bonds pass through digestion and into circulation intact. There are times that they can cause their own problems, which I will go into in much more detail in the next chapter. For now, I have the least to say about these dietary sulfurs because they are the least impacted by the digestive enzymes of sulfur metabolism.

Sulfur-Fixing Bacteria (SFB)

Also called sulfur *reducing* bacteria, these unique kinds of bacteria can use sulfur for energy production in a way very similar to how we use oxygen for our own energy production. Many of these SFB are normal inhabitants of the digestive tract, though in small quantities.

The presence and quantity of these SFB are among one of the most important aspects of sulfur metabolism, at least when it comes to the health issues that sulfur can cause. Figure 4 at the beginning of this chapter illustrates that the SFB generate two primary "waste products": H_2S and SO_3. Those are generated in the sulfation pathway as well, but the SFB production will be of special interest. I put that in quotes because, when it comes to cells, virtually every "waste" has an important use in a different context.

Here is a list of some of the most common SFB:

Helicobacter pylori	Enterobacter spp.
Desulfovibrio spp.	Bilophila wadsworthia
Campylobacter jejuni	Staphylococcus aureus
Escherichia coli	Streptococcus anginosus
Clostridium spp.	Klebsiella spp.

Table 1. Common Sulfur-fixing Bacteria; spp = species

These and other bacteria can use a wide variety of dietary sulfur compounds for their needs. Using enzymes specific for the job, they harvest the sulfur coming through and put it to use in their energy production, with bacterial H_2S and SO_3 being the waste equivalent of the carbon dioxide we generate as we use oxygen for our own energy production.

Because elevated levels of these bacteria are commonly found in individuals with gastrointestinal symptoms, I will have a lot to say about them in the next chapter. For now the key point is that these bacteria use dietary sulfur for their energy, cranking out H_2S and SO_3 in the process.

The more bacteria there are, the more H_2S and SO_3 is made. I suspect you can see where this is going.

There is an important footnote to the sulfur supply used by the SFB. I stated in Chapter 1 that the sulfur in our bodies comes almost entirely from dietary sulfur. That's true, but it's not the whole story. Once sulfur is in the body it can be recycled, and in fact our bodies are very efficient at recycling sulfur. One of the most prominent ways is through the activity of these same SFB in our guts. There are two primary sources of recycled sulfur for those bacteria:

1. Sulfomucins—This is more commonly called mucus, the slimy stuff that covers our membranes from our mouth and nose all the way through the length of the tube. Mucus owes its sticky, stringy texture in large part to the sulfur compounds embedded within it. As mucus is sloughed off the lining and moves through the digestive tract, there are specific types of SFB that extract the sulfur for their energy needs, and of course generate some SO_3 and H_2S in the process.

2. Bile—Formed in the liver and stored in the gallbladder, bile is secreted into the digestive tract to aid in the breakdown and absorption of dietary fat. Bile also contains sulfur in the form of the amino acid taurine that was mentioned earlier. As bile enters the digestive tract, SFB can extract the sulfur from taurine and put it to use for energy.

As you can see, there is plenty of sulfur available for these SFB to pick from, which means there is ample opportunity to produce excess H_2S and SO_3 molecules.

So far, referring back to Figure 2, we've gone as far as generating three key substances: H_2S, SO_3, and inorganic sulfate, SO_4. Keep in mind the lesson from Chapter 1: Our bodies need a constant and large supply of sulfate to do all the things that need to be done. If we continue along this pathway, we need to convert a large amount of these three byprod-ucts into organic sulfate, technically known as 3'-phosphoadenosine-5'-phosphosulfate, or PAPS. For the bulk of functions that sulfate plays in the body, it is PAPS that is involved, not inorganic sulfate. We won't go far into that chemistry, because it isn't particularly important for our story. However, you need to remember that all future references to PAPS is a reference to the active form of sulfate.

So, picking things up where Figure 2 left off, where SO_3 and H_2S had been generated in the process of getting dietary sulfur transformed into inorganic sulfate, here's the flow:

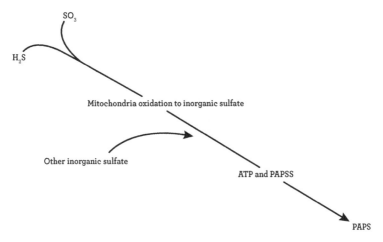

Figure 6. Generation of Activated Sulfate, PAPS

Now let's unpack this one a bit. H_2S and SO_3 can be directly converted to inorganic sulfate in lots of places throughout the body. In fact, this is going to be very important to our story later on, because H_2S and SO_3 are in essence a backup supply of sulfate.

Mitochondrial oxidation of $H_2S > SO_3 > SO_4$

The mitochondria of a cell is where most of the energy your body needs to function is produced. It is where the oxygen you breathe ultimately has to end up in order for that energy to be created. H_2S is produced within the mitochondria, and in fact it plays a central role in facilitating energy production.[5] Remember that H_2S is a gas, so H_2S produced elsewhere passes easily into cells and then into mitochondria. It passes through cell membranes even more easily than does water, which unlike H_2S requires a channel called an aquaporin to get across.[6] Inside the mitochondria the process for converting H_2S to SO_3 is known as "oxidation," and is accomplished by yet another enzyme specifically for this purpose called sulfide quinone oxidoreductase (SQO).[7] The SUOX enzyme

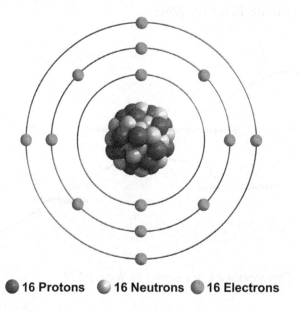

16 Protons **16 Neutrons** **16 Electrons**

Figure 7. Sulfur atom

5 Szabo, Csaba, et al. "Regulation of mitochondrial bioenergetic function by hydrogen sulfide. Part I. Biochemical and physiological mechanisms." *British Journal of Pharmacology* 171.8 (2014): 2099-2122.

6 John C. Mathai, et al. "No facilitator required for membrane transport of hydrogen sulfide." *Proceedings of the National Academy of Sciences* 106.39 (2009): 16633-16638.

7 Michael R. Jackson, Scott L. Melideo, and Marilyn Schuman Jorns. "Human sulfide: quinone oxidoreductase catalyzes the first step in hydrogen sulfide metabolism and produces a sulfane sulfur metabolite." *Biochemistry* 51.34 (2012): 6804-6815.

mentioned earlier, also present in the mitochondria, then oxidizes a portion of that newly formed SO_3 to SO_4.[8]

In the image of a sulfur atom on the previous page, notice those gray dots in the outermost circle around the central sulfur nucleus. Each represents an electron, and oxidation is simply the process of giving those electrons away. It just so happens that oxygen is happy to accept them; thus, the sulfur is oxidized in the process of gathering up oxygens that use its electrons. Again, the detailed chemistry is not necessary to understand. Just keep in mind that oxidation can happen within virtually every cell of your body and is a way of generating inorganic sulfate "locally" when the systemic supply of sulfate runs low. H_2S and SO_3 are the raw materials used to generate more inorganic sulfate.

CoQ10, SQO, and H2S Detoxification

Enzymes almost always need cofactors to be present for them to work. For the SQO enzyme to work it needs coenzyme Q10. Without adequate amounts the SQO enzyme slows down. It is just another way that H2S can end up in excess when key nutrients are deficient.

Other Inorganic Sulfate

This is the next entry into the flow in Figure 5. It brings back into the picture the final product we saw in Figure 4. There, dietary sulfur came in and was converted to various substances, and some of it all the way to inorganic sulfate. In Figure 5 that same pool of inorganic sulfate is simply continuing on its pathway to becoming activated sulfate, PAPS. It joins the pool of inorganic sulfate that was generated via oxidation of H_2S and SO_3, as described above.

---

8 Ivano Di Meo, Costanza Lamperti, and Valeria Tiranti, "Mitochondrial diseases caused by toxic compound accumulation: from etiopathology to therapeutic approaches." *EMBO Molecular Medicine* 7.10 (2015): 1257-1266.

I want to point out a very important and previously unrecognized source of this inorganic sulfate throughout the body: red blood cells (RBCs). The details around this are far beyond the scope of this book, and in fact have only recently been brought together for the first time in a research review co-authored by Dr. Seneff and me. In it we show there is very good reason to believe that RBCs are a major supplier of H_2S to the body.[9] This process requires glutathione, the master antioxidant discussed in the previous chapter. Vitamin B12 is another key player here. It is no coincidence that deficiencies of either glutathione or vitamin B12 within the RBC lead to significant health problems.[10] [11]

ATP and PAPSS

A final step is to combine a molecule of ATP (adenosine triphosphate) with the inorganic sulfate. This process is carried out by an enzyme called PAPSS (3'-phosphoadenosine 5'-phosphosulfate synthetase). The bulk of PAPSS activity is concentrated in the liver, which is where the inorganic sulfate goes once it leaves the digestive tract. It is interesting to note that there is an 18-fold variation between individuals in the level of PAPSS activity.[12]

This means enormous variation in the efficiency with which different individuals can generate PAPS, an important point I will return to in the next chapter.

We've made it all the way from various forms of dietary sulfur to the activated form of sulfate, PAPS, which the body constantly needs.

9 S. Seneff and G. Nigh, " Sulfate's Critical Role for Maintaining Exclusion Zone Water: Dietary Factors Leading to Deficiencies." Water, (2019), vol 11, 22-42.

10 Sushil K. Jain, "Glutathione and glucose-6-phosphate dehydrogenase deficiency can increase protein glycosylation." Free Radical Biology and Medicine, 24.1 (1998): 197-201.

11 Robert L. Baehner, David G. Nathan, and William B. Castle, "Oxidant injury of caucasian glucose-6-phosphate dehydrogenase—deficient red blood cells by phagocytosing leukocytes during infection." The Journal of Clinical Investigation, 50.12 (1971): 2466-2473.

12 Z.H. Xu, T.C. Wood, A.A. Adjei, and R.M. Weinshilboum, "Human 3'-phosphoadenosine 5'-phosphosulfate synthetase: radiochemical enzymatic assay, biochemical properties, and hepatic variation." Drug Metabolism and Disposition, (2001), 29(2), 172-178.

Now let's take a closer look at some of the most important roles for sulfate in the body. We did a brief review of this in Chapter 1, but I need to expand on that now so the symptoms we go over in Chapter 3 will make more sense.

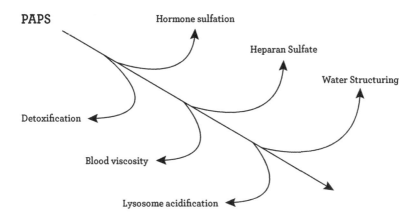

Figure 8. Some roles of sulfate in the body

Detoxification

This is happening primarily in the liver through a process called Phase II detoxification. A set of enzymes called SULTs (sulfotransferases) take a PAPS molecule and attach it to various other substances. These other substances can be solvents, pesticides, herbicides, heavy metals, or other toxins. Once the PAPS is attached, it renders the substance less toxic, and also allows it to be more readily excreted through the urine.

Hormone Sulfation

Again primarily in the liver, this involves the same family of SULT enzymes, only this time the recipient of the PAPS is a hormone: estrogen, testosterone, progesterone, and many others. As discussed in Chapter 1, these hormones act as shuttles, distributing PAPS throughout the body, and the attached PAPS prevents the hormone from being active until the PAPS is removed at the destination cell.

Heparan Sulfate

In Chapter 1 we covered the importance of sulfate for connective tissue. Now we give a more complete accounting of that. Heparan sulfate (HS) is built into the long molecules that make up connective tissue. Think of a single fiber of connective tissue as a Christmas tree, and HS molecules are the bulbs hanging from each heavily decorated branch. Remember that these trees stand like a thick forest covering cells and linings and basically every surface within the body. To carry this analogy further, there are two primary types of trees that make up connective tissue, called glucosamine and chondroitin. There are a few others, but they are modifications of glucosamine. Both primary types take on their functional role within connective tissue only after being sulfated by HS. In fact, it has been shown that when the level of inorganic sulfate in the body is reduced, it reduces PAPS production, and that decreases synthesis of glucosamine and chondroitin.[13] Heparan sulfate supplies the sulfate needed to build strong connective tissue.

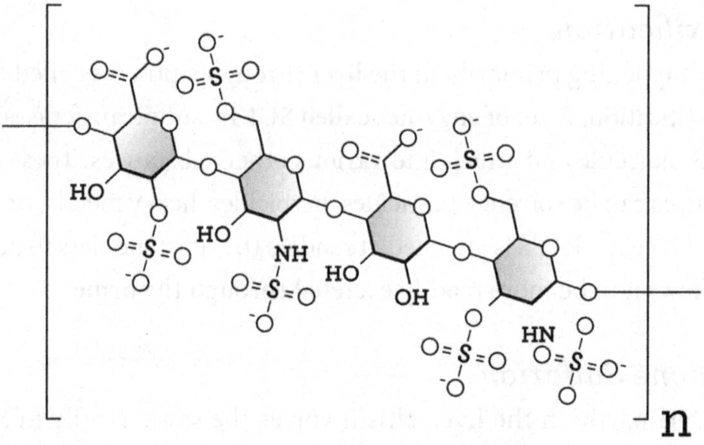

Figure 9. Heparan Sulfate

---

13 C.L. Deal and R.W. Moskowitz, "Nutraceuticals as therapeutic agents in osteoarthritis: the role of glucosamine, chondroitin sulfate, and collagen hydrolysate." *Rheumatic Disease Clinics of North America (1999)*, 25(2), 379-395.

The final two roles for sulfate, which I alluded to in Chapter 1, are among the most important in terms of maintaining our overall health. These roles are less recognized in the conventional understanding of biological sulfate, which is a major reason why I think symptoms due to sulfur dysregulation have remained unrecognized for as long as they have.

Blood Viscosity

Viscosity is just another name for the "thickness" of a liquid. Maple syrup is more viscous than mineral oil, and mineral oil is more viscous than water. As you might imagine, blood needs to stay within a relatively narrow range of viscosity in order to flow through vessels at the rate it needs to. If blood gets too thin (i.e., it has reduced viscosity), then it can lead to excess bleeding. On the other hand, if blood gets too thick (i.e., it has increased viscosity), then the risk of cardiovascular disease[14] and strokes[15] rises significantly.

Sulfate plays a primary role in regulating the viscosity of the blood. This is because it is a strong kosmotrope (see sidebar, next page), organizing water in its immediate area into a "liquid crystal." In this organized form the viscosity of the water increases. Thus, SO_4 is one of the most important ways that the body regulates the viscosity of our blood.

All of those sulfated hormones and neurotransmitters mentioned earlier—estrogen, testosterone, serotonin, etc.—are commonly considered to be inactive once they have that sulfate attached to them. Another way of thinking about it, though, is that these sulfated molecules contribute to the pool of sulfate in the blood at any given time, thus maintaining appropriate blood viscosity. Once the sulfated hormone has been brought safely inside the target cell, enzymes remove the sulfate from the hormone and put it to any of several uses inside the cell. At the same time

---

14 G.D.O. Lowe, A.J. Lee, A. Rumley, J.F. Price, and F.G.R. Fowkes, "Blood viscosity and risk of cardiovascular events: the Edinburgh Artery Study." *British Journal of Haematology* (1997), 96(1), 168-173.

15 B.M. Coull, N. Beamer, P. De Garmo, G. Sexton, F. Nordt, R. Knox, and G.V. Seaman, "Chronic blood hyperviscosity in subjects with acute stroke, transient ischemic attack, and risk factors for stroke." *Stroke* (1991), 22(2), 162-168.

the hormone it was attached to becomes active and can do its hormone thing within the cell.

It is an elegant system for distributing SO_4 throughout the body and maintaining both the proper level of hormone activity and the proper blood viscosity all at the same time. However, this makes it more apparent that reducing the availability of SO_4 or adding anything else with the same strong kosmotropic effect to the blood will upset this system very badly. And yes, we will look at that in much more detail in Chapter 3.

Kosmotropes and Chaotropes

Several molecules that have a charge, whether positive or negative, have an impact on the water within the fluid they are dissolved in. Some molecules cause the water in the immediate area to become more structured and organized. Called "kosmotropes," they have the effect of increasing the viscosity of water, because organized water is more gel-like and doesn't flow as readily.

Other molecules have the opposite effect on water, causing it to become even less organized and thus decreasing the viscosity of the fluid they are in. These are called "chaotropes." Here, strong kosmotropes are to the left, chaotropes to the right:

$$SO_4^{2-} > HPO_4^{2-} > \text{acetate}^- > Cl^- > NO_3^-$$

As you can see, sulfate is the most powerful kosmotrope in the body, which is why it plays such an important role in regulating the viscosity of the blood. You can also see here that nitrate, NO_3, is the strongest chaotrope. The delicate balancing act these two do with one another will be discussed in more detail in Chapter 3.

Water Structuring Throughout the Body

The second of these lesser-known effects of SO_4 in the body is, in some ways, an extension of the discussion around blood viscosity. Before we can talk about this in detail, though, I need to say a bit more about heparan sulfate. Once you understand more about how it is built, its role in water structuring will be more apparent.

Heparan sulfate (HS) is everywhere in us. It blankets the surface of our cells, covers our mucus membranes, saturates our connective tissue, and is continuously produced by virtually every cell in the body. Each of the repeating units of HS is loaded with six SO_4 molecules attached to it, giving it the most strongly negative charge of any molecule found in our bodies.

I want to reiterate that point because it is crucial. Heparan sulfate imparts a strong negative charge to virtually every surface in our bodies.

HS commonly exists in long repeating units of the molecule pictured in Figure 2. These chains of HS can exist independently and thus serve as a shuttle for moving SO_4 around, both within cells and throughout the body. Long chains of HS can also be attached to other sugars and proteins. It is in the form of these combination molecules—called glycosaminoglycans (GAGs) and proteoglycans (PGs), respectively—that most HS exists in the body.

GAGs and PGs are complex and branching molecules. These are the "Christmas trees" I mentioned before in the section about heparan sulfate. GAGs and PGs are spread over all of our internal surfaces, covering and even extending into cells, making up the bulk of our connective tissue, giving that tissue much of its strength and flexibility. And of course all that HS is not just imparting strength and flexibility, but also lots and lots of negative charge!

Negatively charged surfaces do something unique to water. We touched on this with regard to kosmotropes and chaotropes, but now we're going to extend that concept.

Structure of Proteoglycans

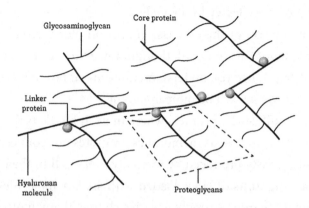

Figure 10. Proteoglycan Structure

An individual sulfate molecule, as noted before, will affect the water in its immediate area. However, when an extended surface is negatively charged, something much more dramatic and long-range happens. The water that abuts a negatively charged surface organizes itself into an ordered layer that extends away from that surface several *million* molecules thick. This layer of water is called an "Exclusion Zone," or EZ for short. It gets this name because as the water builds itself into this ordered layer it excludes almost anything that happens to be dissolved into that water. In other words, the EZ layer of water is *pure water*.

The properties of EZ water are unique, so much so that it has been termed "the fourth phase of water" by University of Washington researcher Dr. Gerald Pollack, who wrote the book of that title.[16] This fourth phase is in addition to the three phases we are more familiar with: solid, liquid, and gas. Dr. Pollack has pioneered the study of EZ water, and now scientists around the world are working to elucidate its unique properties and develop several practical applications, ranging from water purification to energy production and much more.

---

16 G.H. Pollack, The Fourth Phase of Water (2013), Seattle.

There is one particular property of this EZ layer of water that needs to be described in more detail, because it will be very important in Chapter 3. It is common knowledge that the chemical formula for water is H_2O, telling us that for every oxygen molecule there are two hydrogen molecules. However, within the EZ layer water molecules spontaneously form hexagon rings, like six kids on a playground holding hands. In this case, though, the hands are hydrogens.

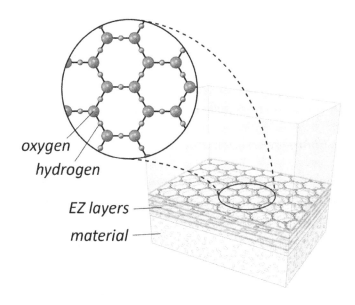

Figure 11. Water structure in the EZ layer

Hydrogens are shared between oxygens, creating an excess of hydrogens, which are exported out of the EZ layer. Since hydrogen has a positive charge, this means that the EZ layer loses some of its positive charge and so takes on a net negative charge. The extra hydrogens accumulate just outside the EZ boundary, creating an excess of positive charge there. When positive and negative charges are maintained close to each other but kept separated, we have a name for that: a battery.

The presence of this "water battery" that is constantly regenerated within our bodies is vital for our health. And those dense negative charges imparted by the SO_4 within heparan sulfate allow for it all to maintain itself effortlessly. It all works just fine—until it doesn't.

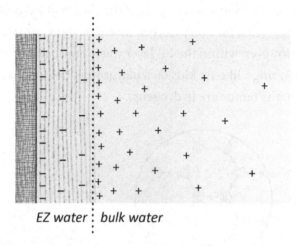

EZ water ┊ bulk water

Figure 12. Charge separation around EZ water

We don't need a laboratory and synthetic materials to create and maintain a negatively charged surface for water to form its EZ layer against. Thanks to heparan sulfate and sulfate in many other forms, virtually our entire inner environment is an extended, negatively charged surface. Since most water in the body is a very short distance from one of these negatively charged sulfated molecules, that means most of the water in our bodies is EZ water. We are, quite literally, a walking water battery!

This chapter has described how sulfur comes into your body, as well as what happens to it once it arrives. We've reviewed some of the key genes and nutrients involved, as well as the role of the SFB in your digestive tract. I've also pointed out two by-products of sulfur metabolism, H_2S and SO_3, which are going to take a central role in the rest of this story. With all that as our background, let's jump into some ways sulfur metabolism can get messed up, and what can happen as a result.

3

Key Players in Sulfur Metabolism

In discussing how sulfur metabolism breaks down, in some ways we're going to begin at the end of the story. I'll start with a detailed description of H_2S and SO_3, explaining what they are supposed to do when things are working well, and what problems arise when either or both are in excess. With that understanding, the various problems that lead to their increased production will make much more sense.

H_2S

Long thought to be a noxious gas, hydrogen sulfide has a characteristic rotten egg smell. Most people can smell hydrogen sulfide in the air even at a concentration as low as 1 part per million. In the 1990s it was discovered that our cells have enzymes that generate H_2S. After a great deal of research on its functions in the body, in 2002 H_2S was proposed to be an important kind of molecule in the body called a "gasotransmitter."[17]

A more familiar and related kind of molecule is a *neuro*transmitter, such as dopamine and serotonin. These chemicals have wide-ranging impacts on our mood, behavior, and memory. Like a neurotransmitter,

---

17 R.U.I. Wang, "Two's company, three's a crowd: can H2S be the third endogenous gaseous transmitter?. *The FASEB Journal* (2002), 16(13), 1792-1798.

a gasotransmitter causes some very specific and important responses in the various cells it interacts with. As a gas, though, it dissolves into the blood and other fluids, and thus has access to virtually all cells and tissues of the body, including the brain and spinal cord.

The amount of H_2S present within any given cell, tissue, or organ is tightly regulated through enzymes that produce it and other enzymes that break it down. When all is working correctly, the list of physiological effects H_2S has in various areas of the body is long, and still growing as research continues. Here are just a few effects that have been identified:[18] [19]

1. It relaxes blood vessels and thereby lowers blood pressure;

2. It can act as an anti-inflammatory agent;

3. It interacts with NMDA receptors in the brain to facilitate memory retention and learning;

4. It plays a role in regulating insulin sensitivity;

5. It facilitates healing of gastric ulcers;

6. It can either stimulate or inhibit cancer cell proliferation, depending on its concentration.

In almost every situation, H_2S can have different effects at different concentrations. For example, at normal levels it will inhibit the proliferation of colon cancer cells. Increase the concentration moderately, and it will stimulate the proliferation of those same cells.

---

18 K. Kashfi, "The role of hydrogen sulfide in health and disease," Biochemical Pharmacology (2018), doi: https://doi.org/10.1016/j.bcp.2018.02.030

19 J.S. Newcomer, N.B. Farber, and J.W. Olney, "NMDA receptor function, memory, and brain aging," *Dialogues in Clinical Neuroscience* (2000), 2(3), 219–232.

Raise the concentration of H_2S higher, and it once again inhibits their proliferation. With these different and opposite effects happening with even modest changes in the concentration of H_2S reaching cells, it is easy to see how symptoms from H_2S can change as well, making them quite confusing and frustrating for those who have to deal with them.

It's clear that H_2S plays a vital role in normal physiology and health. What kinds of problems can arise, though, if H_2S levels become elevated?

1. Most inflammatory bowel diseases, such as irritable bowel syndrome, colitis and Crohn's disease, have been shown to involve excess H_2S within the inflamed bowel wall;[20] [21] [22]

2. Impairment in learning, memory, and reaction time has been reported in workers exposed to moderately elevated levels of hydrogen sulfide in their work environment;[23]

3. Hydrogen sulfide overproduction in the pancreas results in the death of the insulin-producing beta cells;[24]

---

20 K.L. Flannigan, J.G.P. Ferraz, R. Wang, and J.L. Wallace, "Enhanced Synthesis and Diminished Degradation of Hydrogen Sulfide in Experimental Colitis: A Site-Specific, Pro-Resolution Mechanism." *PLoS ONE* (2013), 8(8), e71962. http://doi.org/10.1371/journal.pone.0071962

21 G.Y. Xu, J.H. Winston, M. Shenoy, S. Zhou, J.D. Chen, and P.J. Pasricha, "The endogenous hydrogen sulfide producing enzyme cystathionine-β synthase contributes to visceral hypersensitivity in a rat model of irritable bowel syndrome." *Molecular Pain* (2009), 5, 44. http://doi.org/10.1186/1744-8069-5-44

22 M. Medani, D. Collins, N.G. Docherty, A.W. Baird, P.R. O'Connell, and D.C. Winter, "Emerging role of hydrogen sulfide in colonic physiology and pathophysiology," *Inflammatory Bowel Diseases* (2010), 17(7), 1620-1625.

23 F.L. Guidotti, "Hydrogen sulfide: advances in understanding human toxicity," *International Journal of Toxicology* (2010), 29(6), 569-581.

24 C. Szabo, Roles of hydrogen sulfide in the pathogenesis of diabetes mellitus and its complications," *Antioxidants & Redox Signaling* (2012), 17(1), 68-80.

4. Many cancers, especially colon and ovarian, dramatically increase the local production of H_2S, which drives further cell proliferation and spread.[25]

In fact, there is a long list of symptoms associated with acute, moderately elevated levels of H_2S gas exposure. These include:

eye irritations (conjunctivitis, lacrimation, photophobia), neurological disorders (dizziness, headaches, loss of balance, lack of concentration, recent and long-term memory loss, mood instability, irritability, exhilaration, sleep disturbances), skin symptoms (itching, dryness, and redness), behavior changes (anger, depression, tension, confusion, fatigue, and vigor), general deficits (nausea, libido decrease, gastrointestinal tract upsets, loss of appetite), cardiovascular abnormalities (irregular heart beat or hypotension), and respiratory symptoms (apnea, cough, noncardiogenic pulmonary edema, and cyanosis).[26]

Interestingly, this list encompasses many of the symptoms I see, to a greater or lesser extent, in most of my patients who have sulfur-related symptoms. This particular list describes symptoms in those exposed to 50–100 parts per million of H_2S in the air. This is not a level anyone is going to produce in their cells, not even with the help of SFB. However, the uncanny overlap between these symptoms of acute exposure, and the same symptoms I see clinically in those with disrupted sulfur metabolism, strongly suggests to me that these two are related. I believe that long-term chronic exposure to more moderately elevated H_2S levels

---

25 M.R. Hellmich and C. Szabo, "Hydrogen sulfide and cancer," *Chemistry, Biochemistry and Pharmacology of Hydrogen Sulfide* (2015), (pp. 233-241). Springer, Cham.

26 R. Wang, "Physiological implications of hydrogen sulfide: a whiff exploration that blossomed," *Physiological Reviews* (2012), 92(2), 791-896.

can cause the same set of issues as short-term high exposure, at least in susceptible individuals.

In addition to the low-level chronic exposure, there is one other more extreme manifestation of symptoms that I also believe is related to excess H_2S production, but this time at levels that actually qualify as toxemia, or a systemic toxic exposure.

According to the Agency for Toxic Substances and Disease Registry, symptoms of high-level exposure include "nausea, headaches, delirium, disturbed equilibrium, tremors, convulsions, and skin and eye irritation."[27] I have seen this collection of symptoms, in addition to cold sweats, muscle tetany, burning diarrhea, and visual disturbances, in perhaps half a dozen patients. Without exception these symptoms have come on in the few hours following a large exposure to either dietary or intravenous sulfur-containing substances. I believe some rare individuals who are extremely sensitive to sulfur will generate actual toxic levels of H_2S internally. The very large majority of people will never have to worry about extreme symptoms like this. However, if you have had seemingly random episodes of these types of symptoms that spontaneously resolve in one to two hours, H_2S might be the culprit. These symptoms are much more likely to occur if alcohol is consumed within one to two hours of the sulfur exposure.

Now that you know the good and the bad of H_2S, let's go through the same for its cousin, SO_3.

SO_3

SO_3 is a decidedly different chemical than H_2S. While H_2S has hundreds of publications behind it attesting to beneficial effects in the body, SO_3 has very little such evidence. There is one article, written in Japanese, which suggests it seems to have an anti-inflammatory effect, at least in

---

27 Agency for Toxic Substances and Disease Registry. "Medical Management Guidelines for Hydrogen Sulfide (H_2S)." CAS# 7783-060-4 UN# 1053. https://www.atsdr.cdc.gov/mmg/mmg.asp?id=385&tid=67, accessed 7/1/18.

mice.[28] A second article written in 2005 follows that up, suggesting sulfite is, in fact, generated by immune cells from H_2S as a way of driving the inflammatory process forward, i.e., it is *pro*-inflammatory.[29]

The take-home point is that SO_3 is, for the most part, up to no good. It comes in through our diet as an additive to many kinds of foods, and it is produced internally through the same enzymes and bacteria that generate H_2S. While there is only a tentative and very short list of potential positive effects of SO_3 in the body, the potential negative effects are more extensive:

1. Evidence suggests that dietary sulfite exposure could be carcinogenic;[30]

2. One study, published in 1985, documented dietary sulfite reactions that included "anaphylactic shock, asthmatic attacks, urticaria and angioedema, nausea, abdominal pain and diarrhea, seizures and death";[31]

3. Increased sulfite levels in the body seem to increase histamine production, which can lead to a wide range of symptoms.[32]

That gives you a good picture of these two by-products of sulfur metabolism, and helps you understand why you want to be sure the

---

28 Japanese Journal of Inflammation (May 1999), Vol. 19 No. 3

29 M. Collin and C. Thiemermann, "Hydrogen sulfide and sulfite: novel mediators in the pathophysiology of shock and inflammation," *Shock* (2005), 24(6), 595-596.

30 R.J. Hickey, R.C. Clelland, E.J. Bowers, and D.E. Boyce, "Health effects of atmospheric sulfur dioxide and dietary sulfites: The fallacy of typology," *Archives of Environmental Health: An International Journal* (1976), 31(2), 108-112.

31 W.H. Yang and E.C. Purchase, "Adverse reactions to sulfites. *Canadian Medical Association Journal* (1985), 133(9), 865.

32 C.E. Buckley, H.A. Saltzman, and H.O. Sieker, "The prevalence and degree of sensitivity to ingested sulfites," *Journal of Allergy and Clinical Immunology* (1985), 75(1), 144.

amount of each one in your body is appropriately maintained. Both are intended to exist in quite low levels, and both cause symptoms when those levels rise above their appropriate threshold.

Next we're going to dive deeply into the various ways sulfur metabolism in the body can be disrupted, almost all of which will ultimately lead to excessive levels of H_2S, SO_3, or both. This is where we start moving away from the rather boring physiology and biochemistry, and more into what happens to mess this delicate system up. This section is going to be divided into three large categories: environmental exposures, nutrients, and genes. We briefly mentioned the latter two in Chapter 2. We will cover them here in much more detail, and I will devote a whole chapter to what I believe is the most significant factor of all: a particular toxic exposure.

Nutrients

Molybdenum (Mo)

I mentioned this nutrient in the previous chapter, but I need to say more about it. When it comes to clearing sulfur byproducts from the body, there is just no getting around the importance of molybdenum. This trace mineral is found in several common foods, but in low quantities. Granted, we don't need much to supply our needs, but we also need more under certain circumstances. The average daily intake for adult males and females in the U.S. is about 120 micrograms (mcg). Foods highest in molybdenum are legumes, nuts, asparagus, and whole grains. Dairy products also contain small amounts of Mo, but it is the largest dietary source of the mineral for infants and adolescents because, unfortunately, they consume significantly more dairy than those other molybdenum sources.[33]

Molybdenum is required for the sulfite oxidase enzyme SUOX to function. If for any reason there is not enough Mo around, then SUOX slows down and SO_3 builds up. There are three primary reasons that Mo could be in short supply. First, there could just be too little in the diet, especially with highly processed foods, which have little Mo.

A Thought about Candida

Alcohol isn't the only source of aldehydes that have to be processed by the Mo-dependent enzyme ALDH. Candida, a type of yeast that can overgrow in the digestive tract and elsewhere, also produces aldehydes that have to be metabolized, which requires Mo. This is one reason that individuals with chronic yeast infections can also have issues processing alcohol and also have issues processing sulfur.

A second reason is that Mo could become chelated, or "bound up" by other substances and thus rendered unusable. Dietary copper, for example, will bind to molybdenum, preventing both minerals from being absorbed. This issue of molybdenum being chelated will be discussed in more detail in the toxic exposure chapter to follow. Also, sulfate itself, the very substance SUOX is generating, will decrease molybdenum absorption through something called "feedback inhibition."

The third reason it might not be around for SUOX to use is alcohol intake. Remember the inset text box back in Chapter 2 regarding the overlap between sulfur and

---

33 C.D. Hunt and S.L. Meacham, "Aluminum, boron, calcium, copper, iron, magnesium, manganese, molybdenum, phosphorus, potassium, sodium, and zinc: Concentrations in common Western foods and estimated daily intakes by infants; toddlers; and male and female adolescents, adults and seniors in the United States," *Journal of the American Dietetic Association* (2001), 101(9), 1058-1060.

A Word about Testing

Blood test results are reported along with a "Reference Range" for each result. This reference range is often referred to as the "normal range," which is quite unfortunate.

For example, each time a lab tests uric acid in a blood sample, a dot is put on a graph denoting the result for that patient. After thousands of tests, there is a wide range of dots on that graph, with most clustering toward the center and fewer toward the high and low ends, creating what is called a bell curve.

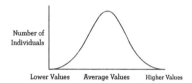

Being at the low (or high) end of the reference range doesn't necessarily mean the result indicates you are healthy. Falling outside the reference range means you are among only 2.5% of people who also tested that low (or high, as the case may be).

One reference laboratory puts the low end of the range for uric acid at 4.0mg/dl for males, and 2.5mg/dl for females. In my practice I consider anything below 4.0 for males and below 3.0 for females to be suggestive of a Mo deficiency.

alcohol? The enzyme needed to process alcohol, ALDH, requires Mo for it to work. If someone drinks heavily, the ALDH enzyme uses up the available Mo, leaving SUOX without. This can happen chronically in alcoholics and can also happen acutely if someone drinks heavily in a single episode. I have unquestionably seen clinically that symptoms related to sulfur are much more likely to show up severely the day after someone drinks more than is typical for them.

A third enzyme that depends upon Mo for its function is xanthine oxidase (XO). XO is not directly relevant to our story about sulfur, but its function gives us a means to test for molybdenum deficiency. This is because XO is responsible for the production of uric acid in the body. Those who suffer from the painful condition called gout will be familiar with uric acid. Gout is caused when uric acid levels get too high, leading to uric acid crystal formation, typically in the joint at the base of the big toe. A gout attack can be excruciatingly painful, commonly described as like walking on broken glass.

Mo's role as a cofactor for XO means uric acid levels can also tell us something about Mo deficiency. Studies have shown that low serum levels of uric acid can be indicative of reduced XO activity, which happens when molybdenum is deficient. In Chapter 6 I will give specifics about supplementation and proper dosing. My clinical experience is that many forms of molybdenum simply don't work well in the body. I don't know why that is, but it is vital that those with true sulfur metabolism issues be supplementing with a form of Mo that works.

Iron (Fe)

Iron is a central player in the building of the SUOX enzyme. SUOX contains a particular kind of chemical group called a "heme" group. You might recognize this in the more familiar "hemoglobin," another heme-containing molecule. Heme is built from what are called pyrrole rings. The image on the following page is a molecule of heme, with the iron buried in the middle of it. At each of the four corners you see a five-sided ring. Those are pyrrole rings. I'm pointing out this much detail because I'll be going over pyrroles even more in the section about environmental toxicities.

When there is not enough iron around, production of heme drops. One effect is that hemoglobin production falls, a condition we all know as iron-deficient anemia. But a lesser-known consequence of low iron is that SUOX production can drop as well since it is another heme-containing enzyme. This means that individuals who are chronically anemic are also at a greater risk of having sulfur-related symptoms.

It seems as if iron deficiency should be easy to address: just supplement with iron. That can work for many, but it fails to work for a strikingly large number of people. There are several reasons this might happen, and we can't go into all of those here. One very important reason, though, is similar to one reason Mo might be deficient: It becomes chelated. Iron can be bound up by substances in the diet, especially if eaten in excess, and iron that is bound up cannot be absorbed or utilized to build heme. Foods containing substances that bind iron and prevent its absorption and utilization include green tea, soy products, and even whole grains. This doesn't mean these shouldn't be eaten, but that they should be eaten separate from foods rich in iron if it is known that you have an iron deficiency.

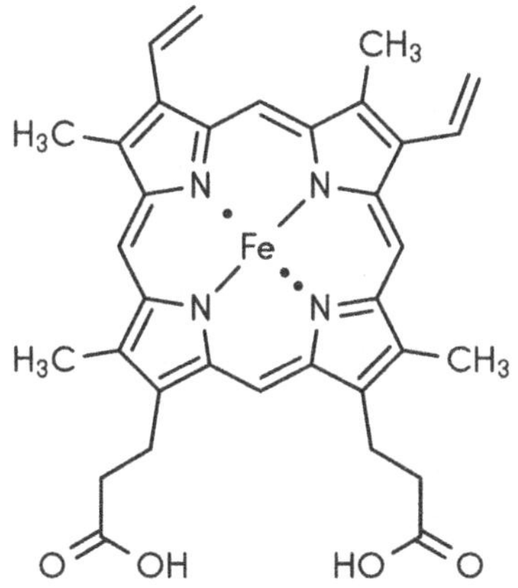

Figure 13. Molecule of hemoglobin

Iron can also become chelated by environmental toxins, rendering it unusable for heme production. Chronic exposure to these chemicals can mean chronic iron binding, which can lead to chronic anemia and chronic sulfur-related symptoms.

A final important point needs to be made about iron. It should never be supplemented unless blood tests have shown that there is an iron deficiency. It is not enough to show that there is anemia, because iron deficiency is only one cause of anemia. Iron is one of the few nutrients that can cause health problems if it is supplemented when it is not needed. Be sure to ask your doctor to run serum iron, ferritin, and total iron binding capacity (TIBC), in addition to a complete blood count, in order to thoroughly assess your iron status.

Hydroxocobalamin (Vitamin B12)

There are three primary forms of vitamin B12. The one we are concerned with is hydroxocobalamin, and all future references to B12 mean that particular form of the vitamin unless otherwise stated. B12 is closely linked to both the methylation cycle, described in the last chapter, and to the cycling of H_2S in the body.

As mentioned in Chapter 2, having sufficient B12 around is necessary to keep the methylation cycle spinning. B12 plays a central role in converting homocysteine into methionine. In this way it works in conjunction with other B vitamins to prevent homocysteine from backing up and spilling too much of the sulfur-containing homocysteine into the sulfation pathway. That is the first valuable role B12 plays in this story.

A second valuable role this nutrient plays is in mitigation of symptoms associated with excess H_2S. The hydroxocobalamin form of vitamin B12 has been shown to dramatically reduce the blood levels of H_2S and a related compound called thiosulfate. It has been proposed that prompt administration of this B12 form be considered in any case of exposure to toxic levels of H_2S.[34]

The third crucial role of B12 in the regulation of H_2S has to do with its activity within red blood cells (RBCs). A little-known role of RBCs is in the regulation of H_2S levels in the body. They take in sulfur compounds

---

34 Y. Fujita, Y. Fujino, M. Onodera, S. Kikuchi, T. Kikkawa, Y. Inoue, and S. Endo, "A fatal case of acute hydrogen sulfide poisoning caused by hydrogen sulfide: hydroxocobalamin therapy for acute hydrogen sulfide poisoning," *Journal of Analytical Toxicology* (2011), 35(2), 119-123.

and oxidize them to H_2S. This process is tightly regulated by two nutrients: B12 and glutathione.

H_2S is produced within the RBC membrane. Once produced, it reacts with oxidized glutathione, which is also produced within the RBC. In this reaction the glutathione gets "reduced" (see sidebar), allowing it to act once again as an antioxidant. Vitamin B12 combines with the reduced glutathione, which feeds back into the enzyme system that allows for more H_2S to be produced.[35] It is an astoundingly elegant system of self-regulation around H_2S production.

We clearly aren't dealing with overtly toxic levels of H_2S in patients with impaired sulfur metabolism. Nevertheless, I test serum B12 levels in most patients, supplement virtually all whom I suspect of having sulfur-related symptoms, and will even prescribe B12 injections for those I feel could use the most support with that nutrient. I will be discussing supplementation more extensively in Chapter 6, and testing of B12 in Chapter 7.

Oxidation and Reduction

We will keep technical talk to a minimum, but here are a few key concepts that are good to keep in mind.

1. To oxidize something is to steal electrons from it.

2. To reduce something is to donate electrons to it.

In the body, generally, to oxidize is more likely to be damaging to health than to reduce. To reduce (chemically speaking) is to *anti*-oxidize. That's why the common knowledge is that antioxidants are healthy for us. Once an antioxidant donates some electrons to "quench" an oxidant, it must have those electrons replaced so that it can do it again.

---

35 S. Seneff and G. Nigh, "Sulfate's Critical Role for Maintaining Exclusion Zone Water: Dietary Factors Leading to Deficiencies." Water Journal, (2019), 4(2), 43-54.

Vitamin B12 can become deficient for a number of reasons, and, in fact, studies have shown that as we age the risk of becoming B12 deficient increases significantly, with some studies showing B12 deficiency in up to 40% of elderly patients tested.[36] Several medications can impair B12 absorption, leading to deficiency. These include the anti-diabetic medication metformin,[37] as well as the class of medications used to treat acid reflux and indigestion, called H2-blockers and proton pump inhibitors.[38] [39]

A second cause of low B12 has to do with how the vitamin is built. B12 is a complicated molecule that contains four pyrrole rings. We already discussed these rings with regard to heme. Anything that interferes with pyrrole ring production is also going to interfere with vitamin B12 production, including a common chemical I will be discussing shortly.

A final way that B12 can become deficient has to do with its mineral cofactor, cobalt. Like molybdenum, cobalt is considered a trace mineral, meaning that only small amounts of it are needed in the diet. Most dietary cobalt is contained in butter and other dairy products and seafood, though whole grains and other foods also have small amounts. Many will be happy to hear that chocolate contains the highest concentration of cobalt of any food. As with molybdenum, if cobalt gets chelated and rendered unusable in the body, then B12 production is compromised.

---

36 C.W. Wong, "Vitamin B12 deficiency in the elderly: is it worth screening," *Hong Kong Med J* (2015), 21(2), 155-64.

37 V.R. Aroda, S.L. Edelstein, R.B. Goldberg, W.C. Knowler, S.M. Marcovina, T.J. Orchard, and J.P. Crandall, "Long-term metformin use and vitamin B12 deficiency in the Diabetes Prevention Program Outcomes Study." *The Journal of Clinical Endocrinology & Metabolism* (2016), 101(4), 1754-1761.

38 T.S. Dharmarajan, M.R. Kanagala, P. Murakonda, A.S. Lebelt, and E.P. Norkus, "Do acid-lowering agents affect vitamin B12 status in older adults?" *Journal of the American Medical Directors Association* (2008), 9(3), 162-167.

39 R.J. Valuck and J.M. Ruscin, "A case-control study on adverse effects: H2 blocker or proton pump inhibitor use and risk of vitamin B12 deficiency in older adults," *Journal of Clinical Epidemiology* (2004), 57(4), 422-428.

There will be several more vitamins and minerals to talk about in Chapter 6, when we go into more detail about supplementation. For now, these three are what I consider the central players in keeping sulfur moving and metabolizing correctly, and these three are perhaps the most at risk of being deficient.

Genes

A few relevant genes were briefly discussed in Chapter 2. That was to accustom you to the idea that, well, we're going to have to talk about genetics, and genetics can be complicated.

Ten years ago there would have been no need for a section about genes related to sulfur metabolism. With the advent of consumer-level genetic testing through companies like 23andme.com and ancestry. com and others, testing for genetic polymorphisms is now easy. In fact, I recommend genetic testing through either of these companies for most of my patients. While I do not use the actual reports those companies generate, I use the raw data files they create of the results to pull out information on specific genes I believe are relevant.

I also want to make a disclaimer about the sulfur genetics, and in fact about genetics in general. I do not believe that genetic polymorphisms are the primary drivers for how people handle sulfur. I think they can play a role, and in rare cases even a central role; but in the large majority of patients I have worked with I find that the genetics bring in an additional, helpful layer of information, but they never tell the whole story about sulfur reactivity. There is one possible exception to that rule, and it's the gene I'll start the discussion with.

SUOX

Unfortunately, genes are often given the same name as the enzyme they code for, so the SUOX gene codes for the SUOX enzyme. Because the SUOX *enzyme* is one of only two routes for sulfites to be broken down and rendered harmless, compromises in the function of the SUOX *gene* are a big deal. And there are polymorphisms in this gene that are exactly that: a big deal. I have only seen polymorphisms in SUOX three times out of hundreds of genetic reports I have reviewed with patients, but in each of those three patients their sulfur-related symptoms were so obvious I didn't even really have to ask much about their history to figure it out.

Types of Polymorphisms

You carry two copies of each gene in your DNA, one copy from each parent. At each nucleotide position along both copies of the gene, one of three situations can occur:

- The nucleotide in that position is the "typical" nucleotide, i.e., there is no polymorphism at that location. Lack of a polymorphism at a position is called "wild type."

- The nucleotide in that position on *one* of your two copies of the gene has a polymorphism. This is called "heterozygous" at that position.

- The nucleotide at that position on *both* copies of the gene contains the polymorphism. This is called "homozygous" at that position.

In the image below, "B" represents the most common nucleotide found at that position, and "b" represents the substituted nucleotide, i.e. the polymorphism.

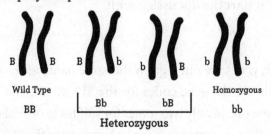

So in addition to the multiple ways nutrients can sabotage the SUOX enzyme function, there is a possibility of a few genetic changes that can further compromise its activity. When polymorphisms are present in the SUOX gene, this is when I'm most aggressive with supplementation, detoxification therapies and the rigorous dietary program that helps to either correct or compensate for these issues.

CBS

This is the one that receives most of the attention in the online discussions about sulfur. Keep in mind from Chapter 2 that CBS sits at the "top" of the sulfation pathway, acting as the door homocysteine must pass through to get out of the methylation cycle and "down" the sulfation pathway. For that reason I'm going to go into it in more detail than the other genes related to sulfur. Ultimately, I find that CBS polymorphisms looked at in isolation can tell us little about how someone handles sulfur.

First, a bit about nomenclature.

Genetic polymorphisms are referred to in a few different ways. I'm going to use the system that is most commonly found in public discussions, which takes the form

[Letter][number][Letter]

The number in the middle indicates the location along a protein where a particular amino acid is found; the first letter represents the amino acid typically found at that spot (also called the "wild type"); and the second letter indicates the switch that can be made as a result of the genetic polymorphism. So, for example, CBS C699T identifies the change whereby, at position #699 along the amino acid sequence of the CBS protein, a cysteine ("C") was switched out for a threonine ("T").

I use that particular example because CBS C699T is the polymorphism that receives the most attention among the sulfur-associated genetics, for reasons I find difficult to justify in the research, and even more difficult to justify based on patients' symptoms. A study looked specifically at this polymorphism and quantified the impact it has on sulfur metabolism. It found that individuals who are heterozygous have modestly increased activity of the enzyme, and slightly more activity when homozygous at the 699 position.[40] Does that translate into clinically meaningful sulfur issues? If other polymorphisms are also present, then I think this can

It's Significant, but is it Meaningful?

When interpreting scientific studies, it is very important to keep in mind the difference between the study outcome's significance, and how clinically meaningful it is.

To illustrate this, imagine a drug given to 1,000 people with high blood pressure. Suppose that 990 of them have a reduction in their blood pressure after being given the drug. That would be a *very significant result*. With 99% of subjects responding to the drug, we can say with certainty that the drug lowers blood pressure.

But suppose that blood pressure was lowered an average of 2 points. Is that clinically meaningful? Not really. There would be virtually no change in any risk by having blood pressure drop by 2 points.

The headline of the newspaper's Health section can truthfully claim that the drug achieved a "highly significant reduction in blood pressure." However, no (ethical) doctor would prescribe the drug, because though the study's findings are significant, they aren't clinically meaningful.

---

40 AÖ Aras, N.Q. Hanson, F. Yang, and M.Y. Tsai, "Influence of 699C→ T and 1080C→ T polymorphisms of the cystathionine β-synthase gene on plasma homocysteine levels," *Clinical Genetics* (2000), 58(6), 455-459.

add fuel to that fire, so to speak, but I have had many patients say they have "the 699 mutation on CBS" as though that in itself is a disease.

In addition to CBS C699T there are a few other polymorphisms in the CBS gene that can either increase or decrease its activity. If increased, it suggests more sulfur will be moving down the sulfation pathway; if decreased, then less. However, CBS polymorphisms have to be looked at in the larger context of nutrition, toxic exposures, and several other genes involved in sulfur metabolism.

Two nutrients to watch with respect to CBS are vitamin B6 and S-adenosylmethionine, better known as SAMe. Both nutrients will speed up the activity of CBS. Therefore, in those with polymorphisms that increase CBS activity, taking either of these nutrients could turn a slight increase in activity into a more dramatic one.

CTH

Cystathionine gamma lyase is not generally discussed as much as CBS, but I find it to be of equal importance. Recall from Chapter 1 that CTH generates H_2S in the process of converting cystathionine to cysteine, and then again when converting cysteine to pyruvate. As with CBS, polymorphisms can happen in CTH to alter its behavior, slowing down the encoded enzyme's activity. In fact, one particular polymorphism, when homozygous, causes an increase in homocysteine equivalent to the increase caused by polymorphisms in the MTHFR gene.[41]

Nutrients to think about with CTH polymorphisms are fish oil and glutathione, both of which will act to speed up the activity of the enzyme.

CDO

Cysteine dioxygenase is, in my opinion, one of the prime genetic players in sulfur dysregulation and ultimately in excess H_2S production. The

---

41 J. Wang, A.M. Huff, J.D. Spence, and R.A. Hegele, "Single nucleotide polymorphism in CTH associated with variation in plasma homocysteine concentration," *Clinical Genetics* (2004), 65(6), 483-486.

CDO enzyme, a product of the CDO gene, converts cysteine to some very important downstream molecules such as taurine and glutathione. It also produces H_2S as part of every reaction. More importantly, when CDO function slows, it pushes more cysteine toward CBS and CTH, dramatically increasing the overall production of H_2S.[42] Polymorphisms in the CDO gene have been shown to slow down enzyme function, thus increasing H_2S and potentially the symptoms related to it.

Hs3St1

This gene produces the enzyme called heparan sulfate (glucosamine) 3-O-sulfotransferase 1 (3-OST-1). It's important to know that this enzyme produces heparan sulfate. If anything happens to slow this enzyme down, the reduced production of heparan sulfate would reasonably be expected to cause a compensatory increase in the production of H_2S to drive sulfate production. It is not an option to go without heparan sulfate, and thus sulfate is also a necessity. We will be returning to this topic in detail in later chapters.

Animal studies in which Hs_3St1 is deleted result in dramatic reduction in body heparan sulfate levels.[43] It is reasonable to think that polymorphisms could reduce those levels as well, and I consider it important to assess this gene with regard to potential sulfate metabolism issues.

PAPSS

A final important enzyme to take into account is 3'-phosphoadenosine 5'-phosphosulfate synthetase, produced by the PAPSS gene. This enzyme passes the final baton in the long relay that races from sulfur to activated sulfate.

---

42 Halina Jurkowska, "Primary hepatocytes from mice lacking cysteine dioxygenase show increased cysteine concentrations and higher rates of metabolism of cysteine to hydrogen sulfide and thiosulfate." *Amino Acids*, 46.5 (2014): 1353-1365.
43 Sassan HajMohammadi, et. al, "Normal levels of anticoagulant heparan sulfate are not essential for normal hemostasis." *The Journal of Clinical Investigation* 111.7 (2003): 989-999.

Once the body has created inorganic sulfate, through whatever means it might come up with to do that, it has to finish the job by activating inorganic sulfate to organic sulfate by hitching two molecules of inorganic sulfate to a single molecule of ATP. This produces 3'-Phosphoadenosine-5'-phosphosulfate, or PAPS. PAPS is the gold the body uses for all sulfation functions in the body.

It is easy to see how anything that might slow down the function of PAPSS would impair that final step of activating sulfate, which would again create a need for alternative routes of production.

To close this section about enzymes related to sulfate production, it is very important to note that two of the five enzymes discussed here have highly conserved amino acids called glycine within their structure (CDO[44] and PAPSS[45]), as does a third enzyme that is vitally important to the movement of sulfate in the body (SULT[46]). If these glycines are replaced by other amino acids, their activity either drops dramatically or halts altogether. As the next chapter will describe in detail, the widespread herbicide glyphosate can and does substitute for glycine within biological proteins. Beyond polymorphisms, this substitution is another potential insult to functional sulfate production.

The next topic, environmental toxicities that impact sulfur metabolism, is so crucial and extensive that I am giving it a full chapter of its own. I believe that unless the environmental issues are adequately addressed, symptoms related to sulfur dysregulation will continue.

---

44 Sheng Ye, et al, "An Insight into the Mechanism of Human Cysteine Dioxygenase KEY ROLES OF THE THIOETHER-BONDED TYROSINE-CYSTEINE COFACTOR." *Journal of Biological Chemistry* 282.5 (2007): 3391-3402.

45 Wilma Oostdijk, et al., "PAPSS2 deficiency causes androgen excess via impaired DHEA sulfation—in vitro and in vivo studies in a family harboring two novel PAPSS2 mutations." *The Journal of Clinical Endocrinology & Metabolism* 100.4 (2015): E672-E680.

46 Katsutoshi Komatsu, et al, "A P-Loop-Related Motif (GxxGxxK) Highly Conserved in Sulfotransferases Is Required for Binding the Activated Sulfate Donor." *Biochemical and Biophysical Research Communications* 204.3 (1994): 1178-1185.

4

Glyphosate and Sulfur

I n this chapter I will be referring to almost every topic we have covered thus far. It is my hope that by the end of this section you will add your voice to the growing chorus calling for a ban on the use of the herbicide called glyphosate, which is the active ingredient in Roundup® and a wide range of other glyphosate-based herbicides (GBH).

Following the discussion about glyphosate I will discuss other potential environmental assaults on proper sulfur metabolism, including other chemicals and a few specific heavy metals. By the end you should have a clear understanding of the risks these substances pose to proper sulfur cycling in the body, and how to assess the relevance of each one to your own health and, for practitioners, that of your patients.

We are going to start this discussion on glyphosate with the basics: what is it, how is it built, and what are the chances of exposure? The answer to each of these will help us unpack its role in disrupting sulfur.

What Is Glyphosate

Glyphosate was originally patented in the early 1960s as a chelating agent, used to remove mineral deposits from commercial pipes and boilers. It wasn't until 1970 that it was discovered to be an herbicide, at which point the chemical company Monsanto patented it as such. Over the subsequent decades, Monsanto developed its genetically modified crops to be resistant to glyphosate's lethal effects, and its Roundup™ product became the most widely used herbicide in the world.

How Is It Built?

Glyphosate is called a glycine analog. This means it is structurally very similar to the amino acid glycine, as you can see from the images below. The circle on the glycine is highlighting a chemical group called a "carboxyl group." Carboxyl groups are kosmotropic, meaning they increase the surface tension and viscosity of water in their area.[47]

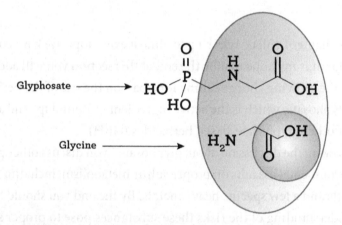

Figure 14. Structure of glyphosate and glycine

As you can see, glyphosate is glycine (large circle) that has a phosphate group added to it. You might recall from the discussion in Chapter 2 that phosphate is the second strongest biological kosmotrope next to sulfate. This means phosphate will impart yet more ordering effect on water in its immediate area, further increasing the viscosity of fluids it passes through. While neither phosphate nor carboxyl groups are as strong as sulfate as kosmotropes, when they are packed into one small molecule, their kosmotropic effect is likely to equal or even exceed that of sulfate.

---

47 D. Al Husseini, "Effects of anions and amino acids on surface tension of water." (2015), Senior Honors Projects, 2010-current. 67. https://commons.lib.jmu.edu/honors201019/67 Accessed 3/13/2020.

Glyphosate's similarity to glycine and its likely strong kosmotropic effect in the body will both be discussed in much greater detail later in this chapter.

Prevalence of Glyphosate

In the United States, the equivalent of over 60 Olympic-sized swimming pools filled with glyphosate are applied to crops and the soil every year. That's 40 *million* pounds of the chemical. When scientists have looked for glyphosate being excreted from healthy adults, they've found it. For example, when 100 adults over the age of 50 had their urine tested for glyphosate between 1993 and 1996, it was found in 12 of the 100 subjects at an average concentration of 0.2mcg/liter. When over 20 years later another 100 over-50 adults were tested, it was found in the urine of *five times as many subjects*, and the average concentration had more than doubled to 0.5mcg/liter.[48]

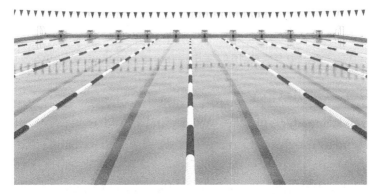

Figure 15. Annual glyphosate use in the US alone would fill 60 Olympic pools.

48 P.J. Mills, I. Kania-Korwel, J. Fagan, L.K. McEvoy, G.A. Laughlin, and E. Barrett-Connor, "Excretion of the herbicide glyphosate in older adults between 1993 and 2016," *JAMA* (2017), 318(16), 1610-1611.

Perhaps you are thinking you can avoid exposure to it by eating organic food. Unfortunately, that's apparently not the case. While people eating predominantly organic food had lower levels of glyphosate in their urine compared to those eating conventionally grown food, they all had it to some extent. It was also found that people with chronic disease have significantly more glyphosate in their urine than do healthy individuals.[49]

The point here is that, given the prevalence of glyphosate use in the United States, we are all probably exposed to it at some level. The government has established limits on the residue concentration that is considered safe on food sold in the U.S. These concentrations vary quite dramatically between different food types, ranging from 0.2 parts per million for avocado up to 200 parts per million for peppermint leaves (see Table 2). A published review of the toxicology data on glyphosate raises significant concern that its toxic effects would likely occur at concentrations much lower than the current allowable limits.[50]

Glyphosate-based herbicides are the most widely used agricultural chemical in the world, although now over a dozen countries have banned its use and sale. Why give so much attention to glyphosate in a book about sulfur metabolism? Because glyphosate seems almost perfectly designed to clog up the sulfur pathways. Let's look at specifics.

Nutrient Depletion

As I've mentioned, glyphosate was originally used as a chelating agent, which binds strongly to various minerals. That's all well and good when those minerals are on the inside of pipes. When those minerals are in your food or traveling through your blood, however, that's very much *not* well and good.

---

49 M. Krüger, P. Schledorn, W. Schrödl, H.W. Hoppe, W. Lutz, and A. Shehata, "Detection of glyphosate residues in animals and humans," *Journal of Environmental & Analytical Toxicology* (2014), 4(2), 1.

50 R. Mesnage, N. Defarge, J.S. De Vendomois, and G.E. Seralini, "Potential toxic effects of glyphosate and its commercial formulations below regulatory limits," *Food and Chemical Toxicology* (2015), 84, 133-153.

Iron

Recall from Chapter 2 that an adult male has an average of only 4 grams of iron in his body, and an adult female has 3.5 grams in hers. That's not much. To put it in perspective, a teaspoon of water weighs about 5 grams. These small amounts of iron have to build every one of the 270 *million*-or-so hemoglobin molecules in each of the 30 *trillion*-or-so red blood cells in an adult, as well as doing all the other things that iron needs to do to maintain health.

Anything that reduces the body's access to iron even slightly can have a dramatic impact on health, and a very direct impact on sulfur metabolism. Reduced access to iron means not only less hemoglobin and the resulting anemia, but less SUOX production. SUOX, you'll recall, is the only way that SO_3 is converted to SO_4. This prevents the symptoms associated with SO_3, while at the same time it supplies the body with much-needed SO_4.

Glyphosate strongly binds to iron,[51] rendering it unavailable for absorption and utilization. In fact it has been observed that food crops sprayed with glyphosate contain less iron than their unsprayed counterparts, and that is due to glyphosate's inhibition of an iron-incorporating enzyme called ferric reductase.[52] This same enzyme is present in the lining of the human digestive tract, and is a first step in the process of utilizing dietary iron.[53] If dietary iron is chelated by dietary glyphosate, this elegant system breaks down. The range of effects this can have in the body is enormous.

---

51 M. McBride and K.H. Kung, "Complexation of glyphosate and related ligands with iron (III)." *Soil Science Society of America Journal* (1989), 53(6), 1668-1673.

52 L. Ozturk, A. Yazici, S. Eker, O. Gokmen, V. Römheld, and I. Cakmak, "Glyphosate inhibition of ferric reductase activity in iron deficient sunflower roots," *New Phytologist* (2008), 177(4), 899-906.

53 A.T. McKie, D. Barrow, G.O. Latunde-Dada, A. Rolfs, G. Sager, E. Mudaly, and T.J. Peters, "An iron-regulated ferric reductase associated with the absorption of dietary iron," *Science* (2001), 291(5509), 1755-1759.

Molybdenum

No studies have looked specifically at glyphosate's chelation of molybdenum. However, we have good reason to believe that it does exactly that. In chemistry, molybdenum belongs to a class of elements called "transition metals." It is well established that glyphosate chelates several other transition metals, binding them quite tightly. Given molybdenum's similarity to these other metals, it makes a strong argument for the possibility that glyphosate chelates molybdenum as well.

If, in fact, glyphosate chelates molybdenum, it is another profound hit on sulfur metabolism. Once again the SUOX enzyme becomes less efficient and less active when molybdenum is scarce, and this impact would spill over onto the other molybdenum-dependent enzymes we've discussed before, ALDH and XO. This impairs detoxification of alcohol and other compounds, and reduces production of uric acid, one of the body's strongest antioxidants. In fact, uric acid has greater antioxidant capacity than an equal amount of vitamin C.[54]

Cobalt and Cobalamin (vitamin B12)

Cobalt is the mineral cofactor buried in the center of cobalamin. As mentioned, cobalamin is required not only for the proper functioning of the methylation cycle, but will also lower the level of H_2S in the blood. A third crucial role for cobalamin in the body has to do with the health of the nervous system. Vitamin B12 is essential for maintaining the myelin sheath that covers nerves and allows signals to transmit through them efficiently. When this vitamin is severely depleted, one of the key symptoms is altered sensations in hands and feet. Clinically, injections of B12 can dramatically improve symptoms of brain fog and fatigue for people who are deficient.

---

54 S.W. Waring, D.J. Webb, and S.R. Maxwell, "Systemic uric acid administration increases serum antioxidant capacity in healthy volunteers," *Journal of Cardiovascular Pharmacology* (2001), 38(3), 365-371.

Glyphosate is known to chelate cobalt, and, in fact, studies show that this is one of the strongest mineral complexes it forms.[55] This means dietary cobalt will bind with dietary glyphosate, preventing its uptake and utilization. This is the first hit glyphosate makes against cobalamin.

The second way glyphosate impacts cobalt, and thus B12, goes back to how cobalamin is built. It is composed of four pyrrole rings. For these rings to be built, first we start with glycine and another molecule called succinyl-CoA. These come together to form a molecule of delta-aminolevulinic acid (ALA) with the help of an enzyme called ALA synthase. Next, two molecules of ALA are combined by an enzyme called ALA dehydratase (ALA-D), which transforms it all into the final pyrrole ring.

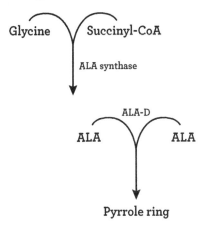

Figure 16. Pyrrole formation

As you might have guessed, glyphosate suppresses the activity of the ALA synthase enzyme, thus inhibiting the production of ALA. The downstream effect is that fewer pyrrole rings are created, which leaves fewer building blocks for the generation of cobalamin, heme, and other molecules that require pyrrole rings. It has been shown that glyphosate causes this reduction in pyrrole synthesis in both plants and animals, and it has been suggested that this is one of its herbicidal mechanisms.[56]

This double hit that glyphosate makes on vitamin B12 is why I believe correcting any potential deficiency is critical in the overall treatment

55 Melissa S. Caetano, et al., "Understanding the inactivation process of organophosphorus herbicides: A DFT study of glyphosate metallic complexes with Zn2+, Ca2+, Mg2+, Cu2+, Co3+, Fe3+, Cr3+, and Al3+." *International Journal of Quantum Chemistry* 112.15 (2012): 2752-2762.

56 L.M. Kitchen, W.W. Witt, and C.E. Rieck, "Inhibition of δ-aminolevulinic acid synthesis by glyphosate," *Weed Science* (1981), 571-577.

program. The inhibition of pyrrole ring production has far-ranging consequences, and ultimately impacts the heme-based SUOX enzyme as well. I will discuss some detoxification therapies I think are a vital part of the program in a later chapter. For now, let's continue with the issue of mineral chelation and its impact on sulfur metabolism.

Abbreviated list of allowable concentrations of glyphosate residue on food sold in the United States.

Commodity	Parts per million
Almond, hulls	25
Aloe vera	0.5
Animal feed, nongrass	400
Artichoke, globe	0.2
Asparagus	0.5
Avocado	0.2
Barley, bran	30
Carrot	5.0
Citrus, dried pulp	1.5
Coffee, bean, green	1.0
Fruit, citrus,	0.50
Nut, pine	1.0
Oilseeds, except canola	40
Okra	0.5
Oregano, Mexican, leaves	2.0
Pea, dry	8.0
Peppermint, tops	200
Quinoa, grain	5.0
Shellfish	3.0
Spearmint, tops	200
Stevia, dried leaves	1.0
Sugarcane, molasses	30
Sweet potato	3.0
Tea, instant	7.0
Teff, grain	5.0

Table 2. Glyphosate Residue Alowable on Common Foods in the US

It is important to note that the concentrations listed in this table are expressed in parts per million (ppm). A concentration of 0.2ppm is the equivalent of 200 parts per billion (ppb). Toxicity studies have noted detrimental effects from exposures at concentrations far lower than ppm, and even at concentrations as low as parts per trillion. A concentration of 0.2ppm is the equivalent of 200,000 parts per trillion! See footnote 37.

Zinc

Zinc is one of the most common mineral cofactors for enzymes in the body. In fact, the ALA-D enzyme just discussed requires zinc as a cofactor. Another extremely important enzyme that requires zinc is called nitric oxide synthase (NOS). This enzyme is best known for doing just what the name suggests: It synthesizes nitric oxide (NO), an extremely important signaling molecule in the body.

A lesser-known role for this enzyme has been proposed by Dr. Stephanie Seneff of MIT and her co-authors. They make a strong case, with quite extensive evidence in support, that NOS switches between making NO during the night and making SO_4 during the day when the sun can provide some extra oxidizing power.[57]

Glyphosate binds to zinc stronger than any other mineral,[58] though one study found the strength it binds to zinc was second to copper.[59] As a result of this, it is likely that the prevalence of zinc deficiency worldwide

57 S. Seneff, A. Lauritzen, R. Davidson, and L. Lentz-Marino, "Is endothelial nitric oxide synthase a moonlighting protein whose day job is cholesterol sulfate synthesis? Implications for cholesterol transport, diabetes and cardiovascular disease," *Entropy* (2012), 14(12), 2492-2530.

58 Melissa S. Caetano, et al, "Understanding the inactivation process of organophosphorus herbicides: A DFT study of glyphosate metallic complexes with Zn2+, Ca2+, Mg2+, Cu2+, Co3+, Fe3+, Cr3+, and Al3+." *International Journal of Quantum Chemistry* 112.15 (2012): 2752-2762.

59 H.L. Madsen, H.H. Christensen, and C. Gottlieb-Petersen, "Stability Constants of Copper (II), Zinc, Manganesefll), Calcium, and Magnesium Complexes of N—(Phosphonomethyl) glycine (Glyphosate)," *Acta Chem. Scand. A.* (1978), 32(1).

is underestimated, because those estimates primarily look at the levels of dietary zinc intake. When glyphosate is present in the diet, it may very well bind up at least some of that dietary zinc and prevent it from being absorbed.

Zinc has hundreds of important functions in the body, from supporting immune cell function to playing a central role in the body's antioxidant system. For our purposes, though, glyphosate's chelation of zinc needed for ALA and NOS activity would be expected to add another insult to the injury of impaired sulfate production.

I could go on and on about the minerals chelated by glyphosate and their impact on health, but let's turn our attention to its impact on sulfate production in the gut. That is where the bulk of the damage is happening, and also where the body's adaptation to the impairment rears its ugly and very symptomatic head.

Glyphosate and Dysbiosis

How does glyphosate lead to imbalances in the gut? Oh, let me count the ways. The details of what I'm going to summarize in this section, unless otherwise noted, are reviewed in a 2017 paper by Seneff and colleagues.[60]

Bacteria in the gut can either "assimilate" sulfur into sulfate, or they can "dissimilate" sulfur primarily into H_2S, but also some SO_3. As fate would have it, glyphosate suppresses the assimilatory enzymes and stimulates the dissimilatory enzymes, thus shifting the balance away from sulfate and toward H_2S and SO_3. This is one important shift. But the SFB that we discussed in Chapter 2 don't just start overgrowing on their own. Normally, their growth is restrained by the healthy bacteria that keep them crowded out. However, if glyphosate preferentially inhibits the growth of the healthy bacteria, then we have problems. And yes, we have problems.

---

60 S. Seneff, N.J. Causton, G.L. Nigh, G. Koenig, and D. Avalon, "Can glyphosate's disruption of the gut microbiome and induction of sulfate deficiency explain the epidemic in gout and associated diseases in the industrialized world?" *Journal of Biological Physics and Chemistry* (2017), 17(2), 53-76.

Most people are aware of Lactobacillus as a type of bacteria important for health. Lactobacillus species are unique in their dependence on the mineral manganese (Mn) for their growth and reproduction. Without access to sufficient amounts of Mn, Lactobacillus species die off and can be replaced by the kinds of bacteria that aren't supposed to be growing in excess, like the SFB. Any guesses what glyphosate does here? Yes, it chelates Mn, preventing its utilization by Lactobacilli and the rest of the body.[61]

In addition to creating the environment for the overgrowth of the bacteria that generate H_2S and SO_3, glyphosate also inhibits SO_4 itself from being generated by other bacteria in our digestive tract. And if those bacteria aren't making it, it puts an even greater demand on our own cells to supply it.

For example, *E. coli* use an enzyme called PAPS reductase to generate PAPS (organic and activated sulfate) from dietary sulfur, then use PAPS to build the essential amino acid methionine. Humans cannot make methionine in their own cells, so must take it in through their diet and/or rely upon *E. coli* and other, healthy gut bacteria to make it. Glyphosate, though, suppresses PAPS reductase in *E. coli*, preventing them from generating sulfate needed for methionine synthesis. Since methionine is essential for its survival, inhibiting PAPS reductase further contributes to the imbalances that allow for the proliferation of the SFB.

A final and potentially catastrophic disruption of the normal gut bacteria population arises due to glyphosate's property of being a kosmotrope like sulfate. Keep in mind that kosmotropes structure water in their local area, and thus add viscosity to blood when they move through it. Essentially all nutrients passing through the digestive tract, once they move across the intestinal wall and into the blood, head first through the portal vein toward the liver for initial processing. Under normal

---

61 Mark L. Bernards, et al., "Glyphosate interaction with manganese in tank mixtures and its effect on glyphosate absorption and translocation." *Weed Science* 53.6 (2005): 787-794.

conditions, sulfate generated from dietary sources through the actions of various enzymes including SUOX move through the portal vein to the liver as well, where the sulfate is activated to PAPS, then used by SULT enzymes for detoxification or sulfation of hormones and other molecules.

As this sulfate moves through the portal vein, it is imparting its kosmotropic effect on that blood, increasing its viscosity. What happens, then, if dietary glyphosate intrudes upon this system? Remember that it has two moderately strong kosmotropic chemical groups in its structure, a carboxyl group and a phosphate. Because of these, glyphosate will increase the viscosity of the blood in the portal vein and beyond, and that is a dangerous scenario. Increased blood viscosity is linked to a wide range of diseases.

One possible way the body can get around this excess portal vein viscosity in the context of chronic glyphosate exposure is to produce compounds that mitigate sulfate's kosmotropic effects. This can be done with what are called are phenolic compounds, and they are produced predominantly by the types of bacteria that overgrow when dysbiosis is present. The sulfate that is produced in the digestive tract can be attached to one of these phenols, moved safely through the portal vein, then enzymes in the liver can harvest the sulfate from the phenol and put it to use.

The details of how this can happen are reviewed by Samsel and Seneff (2013).[62] It is speculative, to be sure, but I think it helps to solve a mystery that has plagued doctors and patients alike over the years when it comes to treating digestive symptoms: Even after a "successful" treatment, symptoms very often return. I think a combination of all these factors—mineral chelation, vitamin depletion, enzyme inhibition, suppression of healthy bacteria, augmentation of H_2S and SO_3 production, and impaired sulfate transport through the portal vein—lead to one very interesting possibility: the "dysbiosis" induced by glyphosate is in some

---

62 A. Samsel and S. Seneff, "Glyphosate's suppression of cytochrome P450 enzymes and amino acid biosynthesis by the gut microbiome: pathways to modern diseases," *Entropy* (2013), 15(4), 1416-1463.

ways an *adaptation*. The "bad" bacteria act locally in the gut to facilitate sulfate transport to the liver via bacterial phenols, while also producing the H_2S and SO_3 needed to distribute systemically to be converted to SO_4 wherever it is needed.

I'll be giving that thought more consideration in Chapter 6, where I focus in on the treatment process. I'll give you a hint about the implications of this, though: If those bacteria are there to keep us supplied with sulfate, then simply getting rid of them will never be a good long-term solution to symptoms.

Let's turn now to one final way in which glyphosate intrudes into our normal sulfur pathways. As with other issues like nutrient depletion and enzyme inhibition, I'll focus on the impact on sulfur here, but the potential harmful consequences of what I'll discuss next are still not fully realized.

Glycine Substitution

At the beginning of this chapter I noted that glyphosate is a glycine analog, meaning that its chemical structure is very similar to the amino acid glycine. This is a big deal, because molecules that *look* similar can be treated by the body *as if they were the same thing*. Unfortunately, there is good reason to think that when the cells of our body encounter glyphosate, they treat it as though it is actually glycine.

Glycine, like every other amino acid, is moved out of the digestive tract and into circulation via a glycine-specific transporter. Actually, there are several of them for glycine, and we'll just call them by their letters: LAT1, LAT2, GLYT1, and GLYT2. These transporters are widely distributed in the human body. They are found throughout the upper and lower digestive tract, from the nose and mouth all the way through to the end.[63] These transporters are also located in the kidneys, stomach,

---

63 G. Tunnicliff, "Membrane glycine transport proteins," *Journal of Biomedical Science* (2003), 10(1), 30-36.

liver, heart, lung and muscle. They can be found in the placenta of pregnant women, within the blood-brain barrier to transport glycine into the brain,[64] and throughout the brain itself to facilitate glycine's role in regulating mood, attention, and much else.

We shouldn't just be worried that glyphosate *could* be mistaken for glycine and transported across these membranes. We should be worried because it *is* transported by these transporters. Studies have shown that glyphosate is transported by the LAT1 and LAT2 transporters, and the authors of one study noted that its transport across the nasal membrane could give glyphosate direct access to the central nervous system.[65] In fact, the GLYT1 and GLYT2 transporters are even more relevant in this regards, because they are transporting directly across the blood-brain barrier.

Additional evidence that glyphosate is being incorporated into proteins as a substitute for glycine comes from a study on soil microbes. Exposing microbes to glyphosate significantly alters their metabolism, slowing down carbohydrate and fat utilization and increasing protein turnover. Since proteins are built and broken down at a faster rate when exposed to glyphosate, it suggests that glyphosate interferes with proper protein construction, leading to the need to break the faulty proteins down shortly after synthesis.[66] This is precisely what would happen if glyphosate were incorporated into a protein during its synthesis, creating a faulty protein.

Yet another study conducted by scientists at Monsanto, reported to the EPA through an internal document but never published in a scientific

64 del Amo, E. M., Urtti, A., & Yliperttula, M. (2008). Pharmacokinetic role of L-type amino acid transporters LAT1 and LAT2," *European Journal of Pharmaceutical Sciences* (2008), 35(3), 161-174.

65 J. Xu, G. Li, Z. Wang, L. Si, S. He, J. Cai, and M.D. Donovan, "The role of L-type amino acid transporters in the uptake of glyphosate across mammalian epithelial tissues," *Chemosphere* (2016), 145, 487-494.

66 M.M. Newman, N. Lorenz, N. Hoilett, N.R. Lee, R.P. Dick, MJ.R. Liles, and J.W. Kloepper, "Changes in rhizosphere bacterial gene expression following glyphosate treatment," *Science of the Total Environment* (2016), 553, 32-41.

journal, found that low levels of radiolabeled glyphosate were taken up into the protein of bluegill sunfish.[67] This strongly suggests that it did so by substituting for glycine in the muscle of those fish.

One final important piece of evidence is from a direct analysis. Anthony Samsel has published extensively on the biological impact of glyphosate. In an unpublished study reported in one of his publications, he tested pharmaceutical-grade trypsin, a pancreatic enzyme, for the presence of glyphosate. To understand why he would do this in the first place, we need to take a detour into the structure of this key enzyme, trypsin.

Trypsin is an enzyme produced in the pancreas. It digests protein, and thus is called a protease. More specifically, its proteolytic (meaning, protein-digesting) activity occurs at a specific amino acid within proteins, an amino acid called serine. As such, trypsin is called a serine protease, and in fact is considered the representative protease in this large class of proteases.

The structure of trypsin is such that it has large "arms" that each pivot around a central point. It is this pivot that allows the enzyme to do what it is supposed to do. That pivotal point in the amino acid sequence of the trypsin protein, as you likely have guessed, is occupied by glycine. In fact, no other amino acid works that position, not even the structurally very similar amino acid alanine.[68] And we can be quite certain that the glycine analogue glyphosate would not work in that position.

Returning to the story, Anthony Samsel had pharmaceutical-grade trypsin tested for the presence of glyphosate. Given that it was pharmaceutical grade, there was no chance of outside contamination. If any glyphosate were to be found in the sample, it would almost certainly have to be contained within the trypsin molecule itself, and if so, it would very

---

67 Archive.epa.gov. (2019). [online] Available at: https://archive.epa.gov/pesticides/chemicalsearch/chemical/foia/web/pdf/103601/103601-269.pdf [Accessed 7 Jul. 2019].

68 L. Gombos, J. Kardos, A. Patthy, P. Medveczky, L. Szilágyi, A. Málnási-Csizmadia, and L. Gráf, "Probing conformational plasticity of the activation domain of trypsin: the role of glycine hinges," *Biochemistry* (2008), 47(6), 1675-1684.

likely be occupying these hinge glycine positions, rendering it much less active as an enzyme. Using three different testing methods, glyphosate was found at a concentration of 62 parts per billion, strongly suggesting a significant degree of substitution.[69]

If our bodies are being tricked into thinking glyphosate is actually glycine, then we need to look at the roles glycine plays in sulfur metabolism to figure out the potential impact of that substitution.

SUOX, again

We have already talked extensively about polymorphisms. These genetic changes can result in one amino acid being substituted for another within a protein. This time we aren't looking to the DNA to explain the amino acid substitution, though. In this scenario the DNA specifies the correct amino acid—glycine—but the cell uses glyphosate in its place. What would happen if that occurred within the sequence of the SUOX enzyme itself? At position 471 in the human SUOX protein there is a glycine that is critical for the function of the enzyme. If, through experimentation, that glycine is replaced with a different amino acid, one with a strong charge, the enzyme loses a great deal of its function.[70] Glyphosate, with its phosphate group added to the glycine, packs a large negative charge, just the kind needed to slow that enzyme down considerably.

Collagen

Another place where substitution for glycine would be enormously problematic is in collagen. Collagen is the most abundant protein in the body, the primary type of connective tissue we have. Recall from Chapter 1 that connective tissue is heavily sulfated. This sulfate, in the form of heparan

---

69 A. Samel and S. Seneff, "Glyphosate pathways to modern diseases VI: Prions, amyloidoses and autoimmune neurological diseases," *J. Biol. Phys. Chem* (2017), 17, 8-32.

70 C. Kisker, H. Schindelin, A. Pacheco, W.A. Wehbi, R.M. Garrett, K.V. Rajagopalan, and D.C. Rees, "Molecular basis of sulfite oxidase deficiency from the structure of sulfite oxidase," *Cell* (1997), 91(7), 973-983.

sulfate, is not only necessary for the integrity of that tissue, but is also necessary for the water-structuring effect. Collagen fibers are very long and are negatively charged by all that heparan sulfate, providing exactly the kind of extended negative surface causing water to order itself into the exclusion zone described in Chapter 2.

The structure of collagen is a triple helix, just three amino acids linked up and braided into long chains of over 1,000 amino acids each. These chains are lined up and bundled and ultimately make up the fabric that holds our cells and bones and the whole structure together.

Glycine, as the smallest of all amino acids, shows up at *every third position* along the collagen chain. Because of its small size, it is the only amino acid that fits into the compact center of the spiraling triple helix. This helix makes a full turn every three amino acids, and you just can't guess which of the three amino acids ends up at that innermost turn. OK, you guessed.

So what happens if, in the process of our cells building these collagen chains, there is glyphosate around? Instead of this nice, compact glycine, there is now that bulky phosphate group stuck on it. The consequence of this for collagen? There are three possibilities.

The first is that it potentially can't be incorporated into the amino acid chain, leaving the helix periodically misshapen due to these occasional "blank" spots where a glycine should be.

A second possibility is that it is incorporated just like glycine, but the phosphate group creates space within the chain at each point it is incorporated, creating a less compact structure which compromises its strength and integrity.

Third, in the patient we should expect to see functional dehydration even when there is adequate water intake. Recall that collagen constitutes an enormous amount of surface area in the body, and the entire extended, highly compact surface of collagen holds water in place as a gel extended away from the collagen surface. If glyphosate substitutes for glycine in collagen, the less compact structure means greater distance between these negative surfaces due to that bulky phosphate side group, thus converting a greater percentage of the water within the collagen matrix into bulk, unstructured water, as opposed to EZ water.

Any, all, or none of these might be taking place. Clinical observation of more people with connective tissue disorders, as well as increasing numbers of people with a peculiar inability to stay hydrated even with ongoing hydration, suggests that these might have a common underlying cause.

Pyrrole rings, again

Recall our earlier discussion about pyrroles and their central position in forming cobalamin, as well as in the formation of heme for production of hemoglobin and heme-based enzymes like SUOX. It might have escaped your notice, in the small graphic on page 32 depicting the chemical pathway of pyrrole synthesis, that glycine is necessary for the first reaction to happen, the one that builds a molecule of ALA from glycine and succinyl-CoA. If replaced by glyphosate it is likely that the bulky phosphate group on glyphosate would prevent the reaction from going forward, adding to the list of ways that glyphosate might inhibit pyrrole ring production and thus inhibit all the downstream products that require pyrroles.

So, we have evidence that glyphosate is, in fact, treated like glycine in the body based upon its transport by glycine transporters, and that it is incorporated into the muscle of fish exposed to it in their water. As of the time of this writing it is speculative whether or not this substitution is happening throughout the human body where glycine is required, or if it is restricted just to the glycine transporter. If it is *just* the transporter, then we know that glyphosate has a way to get out of the digestive tract and into the blood (and placenta). If it is *not* just the transporter but involves substitutions throughout the body, the implications are profound, not just for sulfur metabolism, but for all aspects of our health.

The impact of glyphosate on sulfur metabolism was important enough to merit its own chapter. Now let's move on, though, and return to our review of an interrupted sulfur metabolism. More specifically, in Chapter 5 we are going to look at some symptoms and diseases that can be linked to this broken sulfur metabolism.

5

Sulfur's Many Symptoms

We are going to look into some specific diseases and conditions that can be directly linked with impaired sulfur metabolism, but first I'm going to suggest a new kind of lens though which to view these health issues. Rather than thinking of each condition as a problem to get rid of, I'm going to suggest that we think of each one as due to a lack of adequate sulfate and/or as the body's attempt to fulfill that need. This is not at all how conventional medicine thinks about symptoms. Then again, conventional medicine focuses on symptom management and is not particularly successful when it comes to restoring health in those who are chronically ill.

The theory I'm about to describe is just that: a theory. However, I believe it explains a great deal about why many symptoms and diseases occur, and why those seem to respond so well to therapies that help restore sulfate supplies in the body.

Let's start with an obvious question: If excess levels of H_2S cause symptoms and even diseases, how can that be seen as beneficial or adaptive? The answer to this question brings us back to the body's constant need for sulfate.

If the standard pathways to sulfate generation are slowed or completely blocked due to genetics, environmental toxicities, nutrient deficiencies, or a combination of these, then the body has to figure out a different way to acquire the sulfate it needs. One factor that compounds this issue is congestion within the portal vein. Notice in the figure on the next page that substances (both nutrients and toxins) absorbed throughout the digestive tract ultimately move via the portal vein to the liver. It has been shown that numerous pesticides and herbicides found as residue on food can lead to increased congestion within the portal vein,[71] and we already discussed in the last chapter how glyphosate is uniquely qualified to contribute to that congestion. There are also a number of other conditions that can increase the viscosity of the blood, including dehydration with consequent increased hematocrit,[72] hypofunction of the spleen,[73] low body temperature,[74] [75] and the presence in the blood of inflammatory proteins,[76] among others. Any or all of these could be present in a chronically ill patient.

If you refer to the side bar discussion in Chapter 2 about sulfate's role as a kosmotrope, this will start to come together. Sulfate is, for the most part, generated either at the brush border of the gastrointestinal tract, or in the liver. As touched on in the last chapter, sulfate produced in the gut has to pass through the portal vein to reach the liver. Sulfate in the liver is attached to various molecules, then sent into general circulation.

---

71 M.S.A.E.A. Mosallam, "Cytoxicity of some pesticides in experimental animals" (doctoral dissertation, Mansoura University, 2016). Chicago

72 J.D.J. Kampmann, "Whole-Blood Viscosity, Hematocrit and Plasma Protein in Normal Subjects at Different Ages." *Acta Physiologica Scandinavia* (1971), 81(2), 264-268.

73 M.D. Cappellini, E. Grespi, E. Cassinerio, D. Bignamini, and G. Fiorelli, "Coagulation and splenectomy: an overview." *Annals of the New York Academy of Sciences* (2005), 1054(1), 317-324.

74 R.Y. Chen and S. Chien, "Hemodynamic functions and blood viscosity in surface hypothermia," *American Journal of Physiology-Heart and Circulatory Physiology* (1978), 235(2), H136-H143.

75 Y. Çinar, A.M. Şenyol, and K. Duman, "Blood viscosity and blood pressure: role of temperature and hyperglycemia," *American Journal of Hypertension* (2001), 14(5), 433-438.

76 G.A.M. Pop, D.J. Duncker, M. Gardien, P. Vranckx, S. Versluis, D. Hasan, and C.J. Slager, "The clinical significance of whole blood viscosity in (cardio) vascular medicine," *Netherlands Heart Journal* (2002), 10(12), 512.

Given its kosmotropic properties, increasing the sulfate content of the blood will increase its viscosity.

Human Liver Anatomy

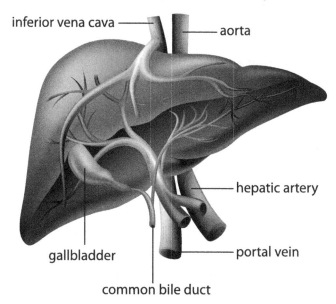

Figure 17. The portal vein is bringing all the blood from the intestines directly to the liver

If toxins, inflammation, low body temperature, dehydration, or other causes of increased blood viscosity are present, then allowing sulfate to travel through the portal vein would "over gel" the blood, increasing the viscosity and adding insult to injury. What's a body to do? After all, sulfate has to be generated constantly, or else the whole system fails.

The most obvious way for a body to work around this problem is to have intestinal bacteria and immune cells produce H_2S! It is not only bacteria, called the "sulfur-fixing bacteria" I discussed in Chapter 2, that produce H_2S in abundance. Many other types of cells, including vascular epithelial cells, smooth muscle cells, neutrophils, lymphocytes, macrophages, and even dorsal root ganglion cells of the brain will generate H_2S when provoked into an inflammatory response.[77] Although this causes many symptoms and even serious health problems if it becomes a chronic state of affairs, those problems are a small price to pay for the benefit of keeping you alive.

In previous chapters I've noted the many routes by which the body generates H_2S continuously. I also noted that some portion of that becomes oxidized to SO_3, then funnels through the SUOX enzyme to become SO_4. This all happens essentially on location at the site where the sulfate is needed. This does away with the need to transport the sulfate through the blood, thus avoiding the viscosity issue. One additional point not mentioned previously about this path from H_2S to SO_4 is that generating SO_4 in this way requires an oxidative environment, and that environment is what inflammation is all about.

To recap, a body unable to generate or distribute SO_4 is faced with a crisis. Overgrowing bacteria that generate H_2S, while also shifting toward an oxidative (i.e., inflammatory) environment locally or systemically, fills the need for SO_4 through a clever, but symptomatic, workaround. Now, let's look at some specific disease processes and how they fit into this model.

Inflammatory bowel disease

This is a category of illnesses that predominantly includes two diseases: Crohn's disease and ulcerative colitis. While these two are different in many ways, they have much in common. Symptoms for both can include abdominal pain, vomiting, diarrhea, rectal bleeding, severe internal cramps/muscle spasms in the region of the pelvis, and weight loss.[78]

---

77 H. Kimura, (Ed.), "Hydrogen sulfide and its therapeutic applications." Springer Science & Business Media, 2013.

78 Wikipedia contributors. (2018, July 17). Inflammatory bowel disease. In Wikipedia, The Free Encyclopedia. Retrieved 02:28, July 23, 2018, from https://en.wikipedia. org/w/index.php?title=Inflammatory_bowel_disease&oldid=850753423

Anemia is also very common to both, due to the impaired iron absorption that happens when the lining of the gut is inflamed.

H_2S has been found to be elevated in the bowel of people diagnosed with both Crohn's disease and ulcerative colitis,[79] and H_2S has been shown to increase the permeability of the digestive mucosa.[80] Glyphosate exposure in particular has been linked to the inflammatory changes in the gut that lead to overgrowth of the sulfur-fixing bacteria, and an adaptive role for this has been described.[81] Therapeutically it has been shown that use of drugs that reduce bacterial production of H_2S improves symptoms of ulcerative colitis.[82]

Clinically it is absolutely clear that a therapeutic diet and nutrients that reduce H_2S production, while at the same time utilizing therapies that support healthy sulfate metabolism, can have a profound beneficial impact on both Crohn's disease and ulcerative colitis. I've witnessed these and other chronic digestive disorders resolve, sometimes in a matter of *days,* by following the low-sulfur protocol I'll be discussing in Chapter 6.

Small intestinal bowel overgrowth (SIBO)

SIBO is a relatively new kid on the block when it comes to digestive disorders. The symptoms related to SIBO are diverse, but there are a few that are almost always present. The primary one is bloating and abdominal distention, which can be severe and is associated with virtually any food eaten. Others include gas, constipation and/or diarrhea, nausea, and an ongoing feeling of

---

79 J. Loubinoux, J.-P. Bronowicki, I.A.C. Pereira, J.-L. Mougenel, A.E. Faou, "Sulfate-reducing bacteria in human feces and their association with inflammatory bowel diseases," *FEMS Microbiol. Ecol.* (2002), 40, 107–112.

80 W. Ng, J. Tonzetich, "Effect of hydrogen sulfide and methyl mercaptan on the permeability of oral mucosa," *J Dent Res* (1984), 63: 994–997.

81 S. Seneff, N.J. Causton, G.L. Nigh, G. Koenig, and D. Avalon, "Can glyphosate's disruption of the gut microbiome and induction of sulfate deficiency explain the epidemic in gout and associated diseases in the industrialized world?" *Journal of Biological Physics and Chemistry* (2017), 17(2), 53-76. See Section 4.3 in particular.

82 W.E.W. Roediger, J. Moore, and W. Babidge, "Colonic sulfide in pathogenesis and treatment of ulcerative colitis," *Digestive Diseases and Sciences* (1997), 42(8), 1571-1579.

bubbles moving around in the upper abdomen. Over time, symptoms typically become systemic and can include fatigue, insomnia (often waking due to bloating or digestive discomfort at night), joint pain, and others. I believe that a whole book could be written just on the role of sulfur dysregulation in the development of SIBO. Here I'll keep it to the basics.

SIBO is diagnostically categorized according to the type of gas that is being overproduced by the intestinal bacteria, specifically those presumed to be residing in the small intestine: hydrogen (H^+), methane (CH_4), and hydrogen sulfide, H_2S. The H^+ and CH_4 types have characteristic symptoms. Treatment focuses on symptom management while using therapies to eradicate the dysbiotic bacteria. This typically involves use of antimicrobials, whether pharmaceutical or botanical. If symptoms of SIBO are present but neither H^+ or CH_4 is positive on the breath test, then a presumptive diagnosis of H_2S-type SIBO is often made.

Recurrence of SIBO symptoms after "successful" antimicrobial treatment is, unfortunately, quite common. Typically, fewer than half of those treated for SIBO are symptom-free several months after stopping treatment.[83] One study of antibiotic therapy found less than 30% reporting "global symptom relief" 30 days after stopping the antibiotic therapy.[84] Clinically I have seen this many times. Patients who have done "successful" antimicrobial therapies *and* who supplemented that with aggressive naturopathic therapies including diet modifications, gut rebuilding protocols, stress reduction therapies, detoxification programs, and much else still often have symptom recurrence upon stopping these therapies.

I believe that sulfur metabolism issues underlie virtually all cases of SIBO, even those testing positive for H^+ and/or CH_4. Further, until the sulfur issue is addressed, there is every reason to think that symptoms

83 M. Bohm, R.M. Siwiec, and J.M. Wo, "Diagnosis and Management of Small Intestinal Bacterial Overgrowth," Nutrition in Clinical Practice (2013), 28(3), 289–299. doi:10.1177/0884533613485882

84 Al Sharara, E. Aoun, H. Abdul-Baki, R. Mounzer, S. Sidani, I. Elhajj, "A randomized double-blind placebo-controlled trial of rifaximin in patients with abdominal bloating and flatulence," *Am J Gastroenterol* (2006), 101: 326–33.

David's Gut

David was 37 years old and diagnosed with hydrogen+ SIBO. He had the classic symptoms of severe bloating and food reactivity, but he also had dizziness, extreme brain fog and fatigue, tingling in his extremities, and more. Based on past successes in treating SIBO as a sulfur problem, I referred him to the nutrition therapist for implementation of the low-sulfur protocol.

My follow-up with him was about two months after starting the protocol. At that time he reported that virtually all of his symptoms were either significantly improved or completely resolved. He still had some digestive symptoms, though the bloating was gone. Brain fog and fatigue were resolved, as was the tingling. The low-sulfur protocol had worked for him far better than others he had tried over his years of symptoms.

---

will return after a "successful" antimicrobial therapy, no matter how well supported with complementary naturopathic therapies. In fact, as I have written about elsewhere,[85] I think that SIBO is much more likely the solution than it is the problem. The real problem, at least in an *unknown large percentage of SIBO cases*, is lack of adequate sulfate production and distribution. SIBO solves this problem, supplying the strong antioxidant H^+, then providing the bacteria that will soak up excess H^+ to produce much-needed H_2S and in more extreme situations

---

85 G. Nigh, *"SIBO as an Adaptation: A Proposed Role for Hydrogen Sulfide,"* *Naturopathic Doctor News and Review* (2019), [online] Ndnr.com. Available at: https://ndnr.com/gastrointestinal/sibo-as-an-adaptation-a-proposed-role-for-hydrogen-sulfide/ [Accessed 8 Jul. 2019].

CH_4 as well. Seen in this light it becomes more understandable why using antimicrobials to simply kill off these bacteria would not be expected to work as a long-term solution.

Dozens of SIBO patients have had dramatic reduction and even complete resolution of their symptoms by utilizing the protocol described in Chapter 6. I am not claiming it to be a universal cure for SIBO, but anyone struggling to find a lasting solution should consider this approach.

Fatigue

Fatigue is one of the most common symptoms any doctor encounters clinically. It is astounding how prevalent it is, and quite rare that a patient describes themselves as having as much energy as they think they should have, given the demands of their day. It also happens to be a prominent symptom in those with sulfur metabolism issues. The reason for this is not particularly mysterious, nor is it a mystery why symptoms often improve upon fixing their sulfur issues.

When our cells are under stress, H_2S production inside the mitochondria increases the energy output. This is a good thing, and is a great example of how cells use H_2S to adapt to changing circumstances.[86] However, as with much in life, too much of a good thing can be bad. When H_2S is in excess it has the opposite effect, inhibiting energy production.[87][88] Thus, fatigue becomes almost an inevitable byproduct of the excess H_2S production, and better energy is an equally probable effect of correcting sulfur metabolism.

---

86 M. Fu, W. Zhang, L. Wu, G. Yang, H. Li, and R. Wang, "Hydrogen sulfide (H2S) metabolism in mitochondria and its regulatory role in energy production," *Proceedings of the National Academy of Sciences* (2012), 109(8), 2943-2948.

87 C.E. Cooper and G.C. Brown, "The inhibition of mitochondrial cytochrome oxidase by the gases carbon monoxide, nitric oxide, hydrogen cyanide and hydrogen sulfide: chemical mechanism and physiological significance," *Journal of Bioenergetics and Biomembranes* (2008), 40(5), 533.

88 K. Modis, C. Coletta, K. Erdelyi, A. Papapetropoulos, and C. Szabo, "Intramitochondrial hydrogen sulfide production by 3-mercaptopyruvate sulfurtransferase maintains mitochondrial electron flow and supports cellular bioenergetics," *The FASEB Journal* (2013), 27(2), 601-611.

Jennifer's Eyes

Jennifer is a 28-year-old woman who presented with, among other health issues, a rash around her eyes that had been present for years. Nothing had worked. Creams might cause it to fade for a bit, but once the cream was stopped, the rash returned. She also had eczema on her hands, but it was the rash on her face that was the most distressing. With Maria's dietary guidance we implemented the low-sulfur protocol after the first visit.

By the time of her return visit the rash had resolved completely, not only around her eyes but also on her hands. Upon reintroducing some of those sulfur foods, the rash promptly returned. The link between the foods and the rash became clear.

Skin conditions

Whenever someone presents to the clinic with chronic skin issues—eczema, psoriasis, dermatitis, pruritis (itching)—the first thought is that sulfur is an underlying issue. It doesn't *always* turn out to be the case, just *almost* always. I wish I had a pile of studies that I could point to that explained this link. Those familiar with homeopathy and the indication of homeopathic sulfur in angry skin conditions will perhaps understand the connection. Those unfamiliar with homeopathic sulfur, or who think homeopathy is bunk, can just take in what I'm saying here: In any red, itchy or painful skin conditions, think about sulfur dysregulation as an underlying cause.

Even people without a complaint of skin conditions will commonly report that their skin is clearer, or have family and friends who comment that they look better after the sulfur protocol.

Menopausal hot flashes

This was an accidental discovery. Perimenopausal women with headaches or gut issues came for treatment for those conditions. They often had hot flashes, but that was an aside during the intake. I implemented the low-sulfur protocol with the intention of addressing their other issues.

On follow-up, I was consistently being told that relentless hot flashes had dramatically reduced or even stopped completely. I recall a patient telling me, with some amazement, that she previously had about 30 hot flashes each day, and these had reduced to zero within a week of starting the protocol.

Resolution of hot flashes is not a guarantee with this protocol, but if I had to make up a number, I'd say at least 90% of women with that symptom going into it have a reduction that is somewhere between dramatic and complete.

Allergies

This was another surprise. The classic signs of seasonal allergies have lots of overlap with sulfur metabolism issues: itchy sensation, redness, and feeling of heat in head and/or skin. For years I would put virtually everyone on a hypoallergenic elimination diet, and it worked (and still works) remarkably well in many cases. However, once the constellation of symptoms related to sulfur issues became apparent, it allowed me to be more targeted with these diets: Many continued to have the elimination diet prescribed for them, while many others would be directed toward the low-sulfur protocol.

Cancer

I have saved this one for last. It is certainly the most speculative, but I also think that compelling evidence exists to suggest that at least some cancers have a close link to sulfur metabolism and its dysregulation. Bear with me on this. I'm not trying to build a rock-solid case for all cancers

Jared's Misery

Jared is a 41-year-old male who presented initially with extreme seasonal allergies. In fact his allergies were prominent most of the year, with only a few months of relief. He had figured out that several foods made his allergies and his fatigue worse and also caused quite severe gastrointestinal distress, but none of his multiple dietary adjustments had given him significant relief. He was taking four Zyrtec every day, in addition to two Benadryl nightly, and that was just to keep himself functional. His diet was reduced to just a few foods, and he was losing significant weight. He told me, "I thought I was going to die." Based on a number of his symptoms, I laid out a supplement program and home therapies (discussed in Chapters 6 and 7), and referred him to Maria to start him on the low-sulfur protocol.

He returned for his next visit three weeks after starting, and his life had completely changed. He was down to one Zyrtec daily and no Benadryl. He had started expanding his diet and was now eating foods he hadn't been able to eat in years. His incessantly runny nose had stopped running, his energy overall was significantly improved, his brain fog had cleared, and some neurological symptoms he was having had resolved as well. We continue to work on expanding his diet even more, but he is happy to have his life back.

being driven by sulfur dysregulation. I'm suggesting a possibility that might be worth considering.

The first important point to keep in mind here is that our bodies have to maintain constant access to sulfate in order to do what they need to do. That's been a dominant theme throughout this book, but it bears repeating. We are eating very little sulfate in our diets. We have to be able to generate it from dietary sulfur in other forms. And if we can't generate sulfate from dietary sulfur, then our bodies have to figure out another way to get it. How might a body generate the sulfate that it needs? Previously I suggested that SIBO, that miserable set of increasingly common digestive symptoms, might be an adaptive response geared toward the generation of hydrogen sulfide and sulfite, H_2S and SO_3. I'm going to refer to those two as "sulfate equivalents," because they can be converted to sulfate within cells.

So now, I present to you another candidate as a source of sulfate equivalents: the tumor. Malignant cells not only generate hydrogen sulfide,[89] [90] that can be oxidized to inorganic sulfate,[91] but they also actually produce both heparan sulfate[92] and those sulfated molecules talked about in Chapter 2, heparan sulfate proteoglycans (HSPGs)[93]

A secondary source of both HSPGs and hydrogen sulfide is necessary if the body is unable to generate adequate amounts of the sulfate

---

89 Csaba Szaboa, Ciro Colettaa, Celia Chaob, Katalin Módisa, Bartosz Szczesnyc, Andreas Papapetropoulosa, and Mark R. Hellmich, "Tumor-derived hydrogen sulfide, produced by cystathionine-β-synthase, stimulates bioenergetics, cell proliferation, and angiogenesis in colon cancer," PNAS vol. 110 no. 30, 12474–12479, doi: 10.1073/pnas.1306241110

90 Csaba Szabo and Mark R Hellmich, "Endogenously produced hydrogen sulfide supports tumor cell growth and proliferation," Cell Cycle 12:18, 2915-2916

91 Emilie Lagouttea, Sabria Mimounb, Mireille Andriamihajab, Catherine Chaumontetb, François Blachierb and Frédéric Bouillauda, "Oxidation of hydrogen sulfide remains a priority in mammalian cells and causes reverse electron transfer in colonocytes," Biochimica et Biophysica Acts (BBA)—Bioenergetics Volume 1797, Issue 8, August 2010, Pages 1500–1511

92 FH Blackhall, CLR Merry, EJ Davies and GC Jayson, "Heparan sulfate proteoglycans and cancer," British Journal of Cancer (2001) 85(8), 1094–1098. doi: 10.1054/ bjoc.2001.2054

93 Ralph D. Sandersona, Yang Yanga, Larry J. Suvab, and Thomas Kellya, "Heparan sulfate proteoglycans and heparanase—partners in osteolytic tumor growth and metastasis," Matrix Biology Volume 23, Issue 6, October 2004, Pages 341–352

it needs to generate them both. It is an odd coincidence that malignant cells increase their production of PAPSS1, the enzyme needed to convert inorganic sulfate to the activated form of sulfate, PAPS.[94] This conversion closes the loop, so to speak, taking us from the tumor-produced H_2S, through the inorganic sulfate intermediate, and ultimately to the essential PAPS the body needs.

It is also interesting to note that all tumors produce large amounts of an enzyme called heparanase. This enzyme splits the heparan sulfate molecule generated in the cancer cell from its carrier molecule, called syndican (S1), another HSPG.[95] Syndican 1 is produced in large quantities by all cancer cells, and it plays a dual role. Production of syndican 1 is associated with suppression of both growth and metastases of a number of types of cancer cells, including prostate,[96] breast,[97] and multiple myeloma cells.[98] In this role it is clearly having a regulating effect on those cells. In fact, cancer cells have been shown to upregulate as many as 16 different genes associated with syndican 1 and HSPG production.[99]

---

94 A.W.Y. Leung, W.H. Dragowski, D. Ricaurte, et al., "3'-Phosphoadenosine 5'-phosphosulfate synthase 1 (PAPSS1) knockdown sensitizes non-small cell lung cancer cells to DNA damaging agents," Oncotarget, 2015;6(19):17161-17177.

95 I. Vlodavsky, M. Elkin, and N. Ilan, "Impact of Heparanase and the Tumor Microenvironment on Cancer Metastasis and Angiogenesis: Basic Aspects and Clinical Applications," Rambam Maimonides Medical Journal, 2011;2(1):e0019.

96 Yunping Hu, et al., "Syndecan-1-dependent suppression of PDK1/Akt/bad signaling by docosahexaenoic acid induces apoptosis in prostate cancer." *Neoplasia* 12.10 (2010): 826-836.

97 Haiguo Sun, et al., "Peroxisome Proliferator-Activated Receptor γ–Mediated Up-regulation of Syndecan-1 by n-3 Fatty Acids Promotes Apoptosis of Human Breast Cancer Cells." *Cancer Research* 68.8 (2008): 2912-2919.

98 Madhav V. Dhodapkar, et al., "Syndecan-1 is a multifunctional regulator of myeloma pathobiology: control of tumor cell survival, growth, and bone cell differentiation." *Blood* 91.8 (1998): 2679-2688.

99 C. Bret, D. Hose, T. Reme, et al., "Expression of genes encoding for proteins involved in heparan sulphate and chondroitin sulphate chain synthesis and modification in normal and malignant plasma cells," British Journal of Haematology. 2009;145(3):350-368. doi:10.1111/j.1365-2141.2009.07633.x.

A Few Words about Biofilm

Biofilms are a blessing and a curse.

In the best of times, the healthy bacteria in the gut produce biofilm that coats the lining of the digestive tract. This film is home to the oodles of healthy bacteria you want hanging out in your gut. The film protects the lining of the gut from inflammation and also from unwanted chemicals or other bugs from getting access directly to the intestinal cells. However, there is always a "however."

In this case, the "however" is that sulfur-fixing bacteria are notorious for creating biofilm, but the biofilm they create is quite difficult to break down, and it does not do anything good in the gut.

Biofilms are produced by several different kinds of bugs. They are like sheets of slime (how's that for an image?) that cover surfaces, providing shelter to the unwanted bacteria. When uninvited, they prevent nutrients from reaching the bloodstream and prevent therapies from hitting their target. Sulfur-fixing bacteria produce very sturdy biofilm, protecting them from even the most aggressive treatment protocols.

Treatment of sulfur metabolism issues can often be derailed by the presence of biofilm. Biofilm treatment is typically done with a broad set of biofilm destroyers, and should address biofilm in both the gut and in the mouth. That smoothness on your teeth upon waking in the morning? Yep, that's biofilm. While some bacterial biofilm is normal and even healthy, some other bacterial biofilm leads to problems.

This isn't true for everyone, and, in fact, prior to my being tuned in to biofilm as an issue, I was still seeing dramatic improvements with the protocol described in this book without biofilm treatment. It's just that, if at first you don't succeed, work with a naturopathic doctor knowledgeable about how to treat biofilm. Once these are out of the way, the rest of the protocol has a much better chance of producing benefits. Anyone with all the symptoms of sulfur issues but who has little or no benefit with the protocol almost certainly needs to do a month or two of biofilm work first.

However, when heparanase starts snipping the heparan sulfate off of the syndican 1 carrier, things turn bad. This causes syndican 1 to become a strong *promoter* of those same characteristics that it once regulated.[100]

Why would it switch roles like this?

Let's imagine a hypothetical situation in which very-early-stage cancers have their own growth-regulating mechanisms built into them. Suppose they show up to contribute to the local and/or systemic supply of sulfate via their production of H_2S and/or HSPGs. Once the deficit of these molecules is addressed, the tumors simply shrink up and disappear. If this were the case, then Stage 1 cancers should be relatively commonplace occurrences, with tumors having a strong tendency to resolve on their own without intervention.

In fact, this is exactly what has been documented. Some researchers have suggested these self-limiting cancers are so common that we should no longer refer to them as early-stage cancer, but rename them as

---

100 Vishnu C. Ramani, et al. "The heparanase/syndecan-1 axis in cancer: mechanisms and therapies." *The FEBS Journal* 280.10 (2013): 2294-2306.

"indolent lesions of epithelial origin," or IDLE.[101] Those authors propose changes in the tumor microenvironment that lead IDLE to switch into pro-growth lesions we associate with cancer.

To that, I'm suggesting insufficient local or systemic sulfate might be yet another trigger. Yes, it's just a hypothesis, but it makes several therapeutic strategies apparent. I will have more on that in Chapter 6. For now I'll point out that one supplement that is a sulfate donor, chondroitin sulfate, has been noted as a potential colorectal cancer preventative supplement,[102] while supplementing with glucosamine for 10+ years substantially reduced occurrence of lung cancer.[103] Supplementation of the sulfate-containing amino acid taurine has also been shown to dramatically reduce several markers in cancer patients while facilitating anti-viral immunity and detoxification.[104]

A final point I'll make in this regard has to do with an enzyme I mentioned in Chapter 3, cysteine dioxygenase (CDO). CDO converts the amino acid cysteine to various other products such as taurine and glutathione. When the gene that produces CDO is impaired, the production of H_2S rises dramatically because cysteine is shunted toward CBS and CTH, both of which lead to H_2S production. Want to take a guess what happens to the CDO enzyme in tumor cells? Its function is

---

101 Laura J. Esserman, et al. "Addressing overdiagnosis and overtreatment in cancer: a prescription for change." *The Lancet Oncology* 15.6 (2014): e234-e242.

102 Gemma Ibáñez-Sanz, et al. "Possible role of chondroitin sulphate and glucosamine for primary prevention of colorectal cancer. Results from the MCC-Spain study." *Scientific Reports* 8.1 (2018): 2040.

103 Theodore M. Brasky, et al. "Use of glucosamine and chondroitin and lung cancer risk in the VITamins And Lifestyle (VITAL) cohort." *Cancer Causes & Control* 22.9 (2011): 1333-1342.

104 Yoshiaki Omura, et al. "Optimal Dose of Vitamin D3 400 IU for Average Adults has A Significant Anti-Cancer Effect, While Widely Used 2000 IU or Higher Promotes Cancer: Marked Reduction of Taurine & 1α, 25 (OH) 2D3 Was Found In Various Cancer Tissues and Oral Intake of Optimal Dose of Taurine 175mg for Average Adults, Rather Than 500mg, Was Found to Be A New Potentially Safe and More Effective Method of Cancer Treatment." *Acupuncture & Electro-Therapeutics Research* 41.1 (2016): 39-60.

significantly suppressed, creating yet another way for those tumor cells to crank out H_2S in high levels.[105]

No matter how you slice it, cancer cells have some very specific modifications to maximize the production of sulfate equivalents.

It's time now to get to the heart of the matter: What does it look like to implement the low-sulfur protocol? The next chapter will give the general guidelines around that process.

---

105 Mariana Brait, et al. "Cysteine dioxygenase 1 is a tumor suppressor gene silenced by promoter methylation in multiple human cancers." *PloS One* 7.9 (2012): e44951.

6

The Basic Protocol

There is no such thing as a general protocol that will work for everyone. Over the course of implementation I commonly adjust nutrients and supportive therapies, and Maria adjusts the dietary component. Not always, but often. That said, there are some elements of the protocol that apply to almost everyone in almost every situation, and the large majority of patients who have sulfur metabolism issues will get substantial symptom relief by implementing these basics. I will go over those now in detail.

Diet

Some will think this is a short list, and others will think it is almost impossibly long. This list will benefit 90% of those with sulfur problems. And it is important to keep in mind, the benefits are not *solely* from the low-sulfur diet *or* from the supporting therapies. The benefit of the whole protocol is much greater than the sum of its parts.

Animal protein is the largest source of dietary sulfur, which comes in the form of the two sulfur-containing amino acids, cysteine and methionine. For this reason, the low-sulfur diet is vegetarian. That said, relatively few patients have become symptomatic again upon reintroduction of meat at the end of the protocol. I believe it is still an important component of this protocol, though, because it reduces the overall quantity of sulfur coming in.

Primary Eliminations and Reactive Foods	
Animal protein	Cauliflower
All dairy	Brussels sprouts
Garlic	Asparagus
Onions	Cabbage
Broccoli	Kale
Eggs	Spinach
Alcohol	

Table 3. Primary Diet Eliminations

Dairy is both a sulfur source and a commonly inflammatory food group. All dairy sources are removed for the duration of the two-week elimination.

Garlic and onions are two of the most reactive types of dietary sulfur, and 100% elimination is critical throughout the protocol. In those patients who are discovered to be reacting to dietary sulfur, probably 80% of them react to garlic, sometimes exclusively or more often in addition to other foods. Garlic is, without question, the most reactive sulfur-containing food we have found.

But wait! Isn't garlic supposed to be a "superfood," one of the healthiest foods we can be eating? Well, maybe. It's complicated. The title of this book didn't single out garlic as the devil for no reason.

There is no question that both epidemiological and intervention studies have found garlic intake to be associated with various health benefits.[106] At the same time, there have been many dozens of patients over the years who get symptom relief with the low-sulfur protocol, and whose symptoms immediately return with the isolated introduction of garlic. So what gives?

I'm not sure, but here's my best guess:

---

106 E. Ginter and V. Simko, "Garlic (Allium sativum L.) and cardiovascular diseases." *Bratislavske Lekarske Listy* 111.8 (2010): 452-456.

Our red blood cells convert the sulfur compounds in garlic into hydrogen sulfide. More specifically, it is deoxygenated hemoglobin that carries out this conversion.[107] This production is enhanced in the presence of glucose, and the endogenous antioxidant glutathione will generate H_2S from those garlic compounds even in the absence of red blood cells. In fact, researchers have suggested that this H_2S production is the primary mechanism through which garlic exerts its beneficial effects.[108] In addition to the other ways that sulfur metabolism can be blocked and excess

---

Lots of Letters: RBCs, H_2S, GSH, and B12

The role of red blood cells (RBCs) in H_2S regulation is quite interesting. Glutathione (GSH) is not only involved in generating H2S, but also in its breakdown. In fact this buildup/breakdown needs to stay in balance, and it requires vitamin B12 to make that happen. If either GSH or B12 are in short supply, H_2S builds up in the RBCs and leaks out into general circulation. And that causes symptoms.

The primary form of B12 in the RBCs is methylcobolamin *except* in vegetarians. They have less of the methyl form and more of the hydroxocobalamin and adenosylcobalamin forms. The take-home is that GSH and B12 have to be adequate to process the H_2S generated in RBCs. If they aren't, expect garlic to cause symptoms. There may be other reasons that garlic causes symptoms, but this is at least one way.

---

107 Joseph Bonaventura, et al. "Allylation of intraerythrocytic hemoglobin by raw garlic extracts." *Journal of Medicinal Food* 13.4 (2010): 943-949.

108 Elizabeth M. Adler, "Vasorelaxation with Garlic? It's a Gas." *Sci. STKE 2007*.413 (2007): tw423-tw423.

H_2S generated, I think that some individuals produce excessive amounts of H_2S from garlic. This would be due to a constellation of issues that might include elevated glucose, chronic infections that might increase glutathione production, reduced overall hemoglobin oxygenation such as in smokers or those with chronic obstructive pulmonary disease (COPD), and possibly even polymorphisms in hemoglobin that lead to up-regulation of this conversion process.

In the end I don't know the reason that garlic is so highly reactive for so many people, but I'm telling you that garlic *is* highly reactive for many people. Obviously many people do fine eating garlic. Many others possibly *think* they do fine, but they are also suffering from symptoms being caused by their intake of garlic. Garlic is, after all, almost impossible to avoid unless you are extremely diligent: it is in most restaurant cooking, it's added to salad dressings, sauces, crackers and other processed foods, and much more. And don't think that eating a little garlic wouldn't be a problem. For those with a garlic issue, even a whisper of garlic can be enough to bring on reactive symptoms such as headaches, body pain, or other issues.

Another food on the elimination list worth discussing is kale. It is a surprisingly reactive food, and I don't fully understand why that is. It is possible that it has to do simply with the quantity of kale that has worked its way into the Western "healthy" diet. I have had many patients who start their day with a smoothie that has a large bundle of kale added. Many restaurants now have kale salads, markets sell kale chips, and greens powders will commonly contain powdered kale leaves among other sulfury greens.

Keep in mind, too, that it wasn't so long ago that these sulfur-containing vegetables were seasonal, so our bodies had the off-season to rest those sulfur pathways. Modern agriculture has brought us the blessing and the curse of year-round access to these sulfur-rich foods. Perhaps we have simply exceeded the capacity of sulfur pathways that were millennia in the making.

The rest of the items on the "avoid" list have been found to be reactive in some people, though less commonly and typically less severely. Nevertheless, these and other sulfur-containing foods are to be eliminated as strictly as possible for two full weeks. At that point introductions begin, and that's where the really interesting things happen.

At the end of two weeks with complete elimination of those foods, we start the one-by-one introductions. Each food is introduced on an every-other-day schedule: Monday, Wednesday, Friday, Sunday, etc. However, there is a caveat to this schedule. If, upon introducing a food a symptom arises, and if that symptom has not resolved completely by the time the next food is to be introduced, then you must wait on the next introduction.

For example, let's say you introduce garlic on Monday, and you get a headache within a few hours. And let's say you still some residual headache through Tuesday and you even wake up Wednesday morning with a low-grade headache. You can't then introduce the next food on Wednesday. You have to wait until the headache resolves completely, which pushes your introduction schedule perhaps to Thursday, Saturday, Monday, etc.

Here is a recommended introduction order. This is modified regularly based upon individual patient history and symptoms, but this order will work fine for a majority of people:

1. Garlic
2. Onion
3. Eggs
4. Kale
5. Broccoli
6. Cabbage
7. Cauliflower
8. Meat (for non-vegetarians; beef or chicken)
9. Asparagus
10. Brussels sprouts
11. Spinach
12. Alcohol
13. Dairy

So the complete elimination period is two weeks, and then there is an additional period of *approximately* four weeks for introductions. I say approximately because the return of symptoms might delay the schedule a bit as I have just explained.

Supplements

The diet alone will get most people only part of the way to symptom relief. There are several nutrients that support sulfur metabolism and the detoxification of hydrogen sulfide and sulfite. No one needs all of them, but pretty much everyone needs a few of them.

Supplements that support this protocol should be thought of in four related and interdependent categories: (1) Those that deal with excess sulfur metabolites such as H_2S and SO_3; (2) Those that manage symptoms of high H_2S and SO_3; (3) Those that help to correct underlying dysbiosis; and (4) Those that help to repair the intestinal inflammation and probable intestinal permeability that results from having this problem. I'll discuss these categories in order, starting with those that deal with the metabolites.

Molybdenum (Mo)

Among those who have read into sulfur metabolism at all, this is probably the most well-known sulfur-supporting supplement, and it is an important one, to be sure. On the route from H_2S to SO_4, there is a necessary stop at SO_3, sulfite. Oddly enough, our body seems not to have come up with a way to oxidize SO_3 directly to SO_4, and instead it has to pass through the enzyme discussed several times already, sulfite oxidase, or SUOX. This enzyme has a Mo atom in its active core, without which the enzyme doesn't work. So, when Mo is in short supply, SUOX might not be able to meet the demand. This is especially true for individuals who happen to be eating a diet that is high in dietary sulfur, which is going to be producing more SO_3 just as a matter of course. This can lead to a backlog of SO_3 and H_2S, both of which are highly symptomatic.

There are lots of molybdenum supplements on the market, and I have tried many of them clinically. There is only one that I use with patients:

What about Antibiotics?

Why not just use antibiotics to kill the bacteria that are generating the H2S? I'm glad you asked.

I mentioned earlier that there are lots of different types of bacteria that can produce H2S in the gut. In addition to all those other effects of H2S that I reviewed, there is one more that helps explain why antibiotics offer only limited or temporary relief for many people.

H2S actually protects bacteria from the action of the antibiotics. So, if for whatever reason, you already have an overgrowth of the SFB, then you are producing H2S in excess. This is protecting all the bacteria from the full killing effect any antibiotic might have.

To get rid of the excess H2S you need to reduce the number of SFB, but antibiotics will be much less effective precisely because of the H2S.

And that is what we call a Catch-22.

Mo Zyme Forte by a company called Biotics. I recommend people chew up the tablets rather than swallowing them whole. It tastes a bit "earthy," and if that's not tolerable then swallowing will work, but chewing it up seems to be more efficacious. The standard dose is to chew up one tablet twice daily with food.

Hydroxocobalamin (vitamin B12)

The role of this nutrient in sulfur metabolism was discussed in Chapter 2. For individuals with the most prominent sulfur-related symptoms, I prescribe this as a series of injections as well as oral dosing. This form of vitamin B12 has been shown to act as an antidote to acute H_2S toxicity.[109] While we are not dealing with acute exposure here, the principle is the same: Hydroxocobalamin will help clear excess levels of H_2S from the blood.

When done as injections, I recommend a series of ten intramuscular injections with 5mg hydroxocobalamin, injections happening every other day. For that larger portion of patients for whom oral supplementation is sufficient, I am using a Biotics product containing 2000mcg (2mg) of hydroxocobalamin per lozenge, called B12-2000, and I recommend 1–2 daily depending on the patient. I am not paid by them to use or advertise their products—they just happen to have some that work really well for sulfur patients.

Flaxseed powder

When dealing with excess H_2S production, one approach is to inhibit the enzymes that are responsible for producing it. That's precisely what flaxseed powder does. It inhibits those two major enzymes involved in H_2S production, CBS and CTH,[110] both discussed in detail in Chapter 2.

The perk here is that flaxseed powder is a great source of dietary soluble fiber, providing some of the prebiotic fuel needed for healthy bacteria to produce much-needed short-chained fatty acids. I typically dose this at 1 tablespoon twice daily sprinkled on food, blended into a smoothie, mixed into (gluten-free) oatmeal, or for the brave, simply stirred into water. Drink that quickly, though, because it will turn the water into a gel before long.

An important side note here is that, for individuals who struggle with constipation, flaxseed powder can be a help or a hindrance. For some, the help is that it keeps them regular. For others, it causes bloating

---

109 Yuji Fujita, et al. "A fatal case of acute hydrogen sulfide poisoning caused by hydrogen sulfide: hydroxocobalamin therapy for acute hydrogen sulfide poisoning." *Journal of Analytical Toxicology* 35.2 (2011): 119-123.

110 Shyamchand Mayengbam, et al. "A Vitamin B-6 Antagonist from Flaxseed Perturbs Amino Acid Metabolism in Moderately Vitamin B-6–Deficient Male Rats–3." *The Journal of Nutrition* 146.1 (2015): 14-20.

and worsens the constipation. If the latter happens even with sufficient water intake, then obviously it is not the right support for this protocol. Sufficient water intake is the amount that leads to the need to urinate approximately every 1.5 to 2 hours throughout the day. This typically works out to drinking, in ounces, ½ body weight (measured in pounds). For example, a 150-lb person should drink 75 oz of water over the course of their waking hours.

Korean Red Ginseng (KRG)

This is another supplement that can inhibit the enzymes that produce H_2S, most specifically the same two enzymes worked on by flaxseed powder: CBS and CTH (the latter is also referred to in studies as CSE).[111] Many people with sulfur issues suffer from fatigue, sometimes quite debilitating. KRG can help with this symptom as well, so it is especially indicated for those individuals. I prescribe it for a minority of patients, but when I do it is usually 1,000mg twice daily with food.

Capsaicin

This is the most widely recognized medicinal constituent of cayenne pepper. This one works on the receptors that are stimulated by H_2S, including both motor[112] and pain[113] receptors. For this reason, I think of it in those situations where patients have abdominal cramping along with bloating, or when pain is a significant symptom anywhere, intestinal or otherwise. I typically prescribe a tincture, 1 dropper 4 times daily in juice. This stuff is hot on your tongue, so don't try it without diluting it,

---

111 Sooyeon Lee, et al. "Korean red ginseng ameliorated experimental pancreatitis through the inhibition of hydrogen sulfide in mice." *Pancreatology* 16.3 (2016): 326-336.

112 Riccardo Patacchini, et al. "Hydrogen sulfide (H2S) stimulates capsaicin-sensitive primary afferent neurons in the rat urinary bladder." *British Journal of Pharmacology* 142.1 (2004): 31–34.

113 Sachiyo Nishimura, et al. "Hydrogen sulfide as a novel mediator for pancreatic pain in rodents." *Gut* (2009).

and even with dilution it can light you up a bit. Use caution. Consider yourself warned.

Bismuth

Why does Pepto-Bismol® work? Because a lot of people have a sulfur problem. As the name suggests, it works because the chemical element bismuth, its active ingredient, binds to H_2S and thus prevents it from going on to cause problems.[114] This can reduce gas production and relieve bloating, but it doesn't alter the bacteria that are producing it in the first place. That's not to say that it is useless. Some people need quick relief from severe bloating. I most commonly prescribe a bismuth-containing supplement when bloating happens at night and interrupts sleep. A bismuth subsalicylate or bismuth citrate supplement (*not* Pepto-Bismol®) can reduce nighttime bloating and thus allow for a more restful sleep.

Probiotics

This one seems to be controversial, especially among those with the diagnosis of SIBO. I side with ancient Greek physician Paracelsus on this one: "The dose is the poison." The flip side of that coin, though, is that the *proper* dose is therapeutic. I recommend a spore-based probiotic to virtually every patient with significant gastrointestinal symptoms, including those with a diagnosis of SIBO. The trick is in the dosing.

I commonly find that we have to start with as little as 1/4 of a capsule (opened up and sprinkled on food), every other day. Some people really are this sensitive. Over time we titrate up the dose, all the while working through the protocol to help sulfur process the way it needs to. It is exceedingly rare that someone simply cannot tolerate any amount of these probiotics. In my own practice I'm using a brand that is only available through a licensed health care practitioner, called MegaSporeBiotic by

---

114 Fabrizis L. Suarez, et al. "Bismuth subsalicylate markedly decreases hydrogen sulfide release in the human colon." *Gastroenterology* 114.5 (1998): 923–929.

Microbiome Labs. For those who can tolerate it well, I will commonly dose it at two capsules once or twice daily with food.

While I think the spore-based probiotics are important, I also believe it is important to supplement with others as well. An ideal probiotic program utilizes the spore-based probiotics at one meal, then another probiotic containing several Lactobacillus and Bifidobacteria species at another meal.

Lemongrass

There are a number of herbs that have the effect of suppressing the growth of the sulfur-fixing bacteria. Lemongrass is the one I prefer, as it seems to work well for most people, and it has a decent taste.

Beyond that, lemongrass has a bevy of other beneficial effects that are often called for with sulfur-sensitive people. It can help with anxiety, depression, and sleep, all issues common to people with sulfur metabolism issues. It is very important that essential oils always be organically sourced. I typically dose this starting with three drops twice daily. This can be mixed into a small amount of juice, or some patients put the drops into capsules and take it that way. Every third day I recommend increasing the dose by one drop per dose up to a maximum of six drops twice daily. A few patients have felt considerably better by going to a much higher dose, but I don't recommend that generally.

Butyrate

I believe butyrate is the most underrated nutrient there is. It is a short-chain fatty acid produced by specific types of beneficial bacteria that are *supposed to* grow in ample quantities in the gut. What could possibly prevent those bacteria from being present in adequate quantities? We could sum it up by saying it's modern life. Medications, stress, alcohol, inflammation, and any number of conditions causing dysbiosis can result in significantly reduced production of butyrate by those gut bacteria.

What everyone should know about short-chain fatty acids (SCFAs)

There are three SCFAs that are important to maintaining health: butyrate, propionate, and acetate. These are produced when dietary soluble fiber, such as oatmeal, flax and chia seeds, beans, apples, and many other foods, are digested by those healthy bacteria.

While butyrate is receiving most of the attention here, the other two are essential for health in their own way. Propionate has been shown to lower cholesterol and reduce inflammation, and acetate is also anti-inflammatory and is involved in energy production within cells.

What's so great about butyrate? Well, lots of things. Butyrate reduces inflammation both in the gut and systemically. Individuals with inflammatory bowel diseases have been shown to be almost universally low in gut butyrate levels.[115] Perhaps even more importantly, butyrate might just be the stuff that gives fiber its anti-cancer benefits by suppressing the cancer-promoting genes in the colon, and activating the cancer-preventing genes in those same cells.[116] Most relevant to this sulfur issue, high levels of H_2S lead to gut inflammation, which leads to a loss of integrity in the gut lining (aka "leaky gut"). Butyrate helps to

---

115 Filip Van Immerseel, et al. "Butyric acid-producing anaerobic bacteria as a novel probiotic treatment approach for inflammatory bowel disease." *Journal of Medical Microbiology* 59.2 (2010): 141–143.

116 Scott J. Bultman, "Molecular pathways: gene–environment interactions regulating dietary fiber induction of proliferation and apoptosis via butyrate for cancer prevention." *Clinical Cancer Research* 20.4 (2014): 799–803.

reestablish the integrity of the gut lining,[117] ultimately making a wide range of foods less reactive.

Butyrate can be dosed quite high, and it is rare that it causes any kind of negative effect, even in sensitive patients. A common dose is 1g twice daily using one of the butyrate salts (calcium or magnesium butyrate). In my practice I'm using either Butyric Cal/Mag by Biotics, EnteroVite by Apex Energetics, or ProButyrate by Tesseract. It just depends on what effect I want to emphasize in the patient. For patients with diarrhea as a predominant symptom, dosing can go as high as 3 grams twice daily with food.

Those are the most important elements of the low-sulfur diet and supplement protocol. Next I will discuss some labs that are important to both assessing and monitoring sulfur issues.

---

117 Luying Peng, et al. "Butyrate enhances the intestinal barrier by facilitating tight junction assembly via activation of AMP-activated protein kinase in Caco-2 cell monolayers." *The Journal of Nutrition* 139.9 (2009): 1619–1625.

7

Helpful Lab Tests

One of the most common questions I am asked is, "Isn't there a test I can do to find out if I have a problem with sulfur?" In short, no, there isn't. Sulfur isn't unique in this way. For instance, I have had dozens of patients who report to me that they feel worse upon eating some particular food, yet food reactivity testing doesn't show those foods to be problems for those people. My suspicion is that this is because excess H_2S is primarily being produced within the cells, so you can't "see" it with a test.

There are a few tests, though, that I believe are valuable when evaluating sulfur issues. None of these tests is unusual, so anyone should be able to ask their doctor to order them. Granted, most conventional doctors are not going to be accustomed to ordering some of these tests, and that is all the more reason to find a naturopathic doctor to work with. These tests will be familiar to them all.

Complete Blood Count (CBC)

Pretty much everyone who has labs at their yearly physical is having a CBC run. The important point is the interpretation. This test is typically used to identify anemia, where low hemoglobin and/or hematocrit (referred to as "H&H" in the biz) signify, by definition, anemia. The key on the CBC is a close reading of how the numbers shift.

1. Total red blood cells (RBCs)—Most labs put the low end of the RBC range around 3.8 million cells per mm^3. Numbers below 4.2 are, I believe, suspicious if other sulfur symptoms are present. Keep in mind that if, as I suspect, RBCs are a primary source of H_2S, an adaptive reduction of RBCs in response to high H_2S generated elsewhere would be expected. Also remember that RBCs are an important source of glutathione production.[118] Both of these roles keep RBCs in the center of proper sulfur metabolism. If RBCs are elevated above the reference range, and if dehydration has been ruled out, consider this as possibly the body's attempt to generate additional H_2S and, subsequently, SO_4.

2. Hemoglobin and hematocrit (H&H)—Levels of these that are below the lab-specified range qualify someone as anemic. However, determining *that* someone is anemic is the easy part; determining *why* is more challenging and depends on the rest of the labs listed here. Hemoglobin plays a direct role in the oxidation of some sulfur compounds, turning them into H_2S, as mentioned previously. Low numbers here mean anemia. High numbers need investigation. Consider dehydration, and also consider compensation to generate more H_2S.

3. Mean Corpuscular Volume (MCV)—I used to put a lot of weight on this one as an indication of vitamin B12 deficiency, but I don't anymore. I notice it, and if it is very elevated—97fL or above—then I consider it important. But I no longer see it as a reliable general marker of vitamin B12 sufficiency. I believe the evidence backs me up on this. Even those who have had very

---

118 Anna Bogdanova and Hans U. Lutz. "Mechanisms tagging senescent red blood cells for clearance in healthy humans." *Frontiers in Physiology* (4) (2013): 387.

dramatically low levels of serum B12 for years can have normal MCV and other values on their CBC.[119]

4. Mean Corpuscular Hemoglobin (MCH)—This is, I believe, a more sensitive marker of vitamin B12 deficiency, and especially when looked at in combination with the MCV and with platelets. Most lab ranges put the upper limit for this value at 32mcg. Research suggests that anything above 30.9 is suggestive of a vitamin B12 deficiency. Further, a ratio of the platelets to MCH is an even more specific way of quantifying deficiencies of both B12 and iron.[120]

These numbers are only to be thought of as supplementary information. They do not accurately identify nutrient issues in and of themselves.

Serum B12

Here's the thing about serum B12: If it is elevated, it could be falsely elevated, but if it is low, it is truly low.

There are lots of reasons that serum B12 might be elevated, the most important being recent B12 intake via injections or supplements, and genetic polymorphisms that prevent the vitamin from getting from the blood and into cells. I test serum B12 on almost all my patients. If they test high, I don't assume they have enough B12 in their cells. If they test low, I assume they definitely need more of this vitamin.

Most lab ranges are 200 to about 900pg/mL. This is a tragic range. If fasting serum B12 is below 650, I assume deficiency. If below 400, I consider it a very significant deficiency. If even close to 200, I treat it very

119 Allen Dong and Stephen C. Scott. "Serum vitamin B12 and blood cell values in vegetarians." *Annals of Nutrition and Metabolism* 26.4 (1982): 209–216.

120 Cengiz Beyan, et al. "The platelet count/mean corpuscular hemoglobin ratio distinguishes combined iron and vitamin B 12 deficiency from uncomplicated iron deficiency." *International Journal of Hematology* 81.4 (2005): 301–303.

aggressively. Individuals with B12 this low are almost always symptomatic: severe fatigue, altered sensation in hands and feet, brain fog, often low blood pressure, and other issues.

High-serum vitamin B12 on labs is largely irrelevant. It can make some conventional doctors nervous, but there is no risk to high-serum B12 and, in fact, it can be valuable diagnostic information, especially in those individuals who have clear signs of vitamin B12 deficiency.

Serum homocysteine

This is probably the most important standard lab test to assess sulfur issues. It is meaningful if either high or low. Again, lab ranges are unreliable. Optimal is 7mmol/L. Elevations above 9 indicate problems, and this is the point at which risks start to rise. Also, it is important to note that an elevation in homocysteine is a more reliable marker of vitamin B12 and/or folate deficiency than any of those CBC parameters like MCV or MCH I discussed previously.[121] Many labs place the upper limit of the reference range for homocysteine at 15, but research suggests an individual could have more than a 33% increased risk of dying due to the effects of elevated homocysteine even though their homocysteine is significantly less than 15.[122]

While I find high homocysteine to be important for its own reasons, I think that low homocysteine is even more relevant when it comes to sulfur. When someone tests below 7 the first question to ask is, "Are you eating a low-protein diet?" If the answer to that is "no," then my suspicion level rises the lower the homocysteine is. Keep in mind that homocysteine sits at the beginning of the sulfation pathways. If conditions are in place to

---

121 M. Haltmayer, T. Mueller, and W. Poelz. "Erythrocyte mean cellular volume and its relation to serum homocysteine, vitamin B12 and folate." *Acta Medica Austriaca* 29.2 (2002): 57–60.
122 Hui-yong Peng, et al. "Elevated homocysteine levels and risk of cardiovascular and all-cause mortality: a meta-analysis of prospective studies." *Journal of Zhejiang University-Science* B 16.1 (2015): 78–86.

draw excess homocysteine down those pathways, then we should expect low homocysteine to correlate with more sulfur symptoms.

In my experience, assuming an adequate protein intake, homocysteine in the 6s is suggestive of sulfur problems. If homocysteine is in the 5s, it is almost certain that there are going to be sulfur problems. I have only once out of many hundreds of tests seen homocysteine below 5, and sulfur was definitely causing symptoms for that patient. I highly recommend homocysteine be checked as a part of standard blood work. If it is high, there is likely a methylation problem that needs to be solved with specific nutrients. Many of those nutrients are *also* critical for proper sulfur metabolism. If it is low, it is probably being drawn "down" the sulfur pathways, lots of H_2S is being generated, and it needs to be solved with the sulfur-based therapies discussed in this book.

GGT (gamma glutamyltransferase)

This marker is highly underrated. It should be run yearly on everyone. The evidence of its utility as a risk factor for many issues is compelling, and I think it gives us some insight into sulfur issues in particular.

Glutathione has been mentioned several times previously. It is a big deal. The standard thinking about the GGT enzyme is that its job is to break glutathione outside the cell down into its constituent parts: glutamine, glycine and cysteine. Once broken down, so the standard story goes, those can get transported into the cell to get reassembled into new glutathione. This model, though, seems unlikely to be the whole story. Why not just transport glutathione across the cell membrane if it is such a critical molecule for cellular health? Maybe the standard story needs some updating.

Dr. Seneff and her co-authors proposed a different role for GGT, one that makes a whole lot more sense. In this model GGT doesn't break down glutathione only to have it rebuilt inside the cell. Instead, if there is a general deficiency of sulfate, GGT breaks down glutathione to liberate the cysteine. Cysteine in the blood can then be acted on enzymatically by CBS, CTH, or CDO to produce H_2S and then, with a little help from oxidation, SO_4.[123]

GGT elevations are associated with increased levels of oxidative stress,[124] which is reflected by the fact that serum antioxidant levels tend to be low when GGT levels are high.[125] I test this enzyme on every patient, and I don't use lab reference ranges, which vary widely from lab to lab. GGT should be 13U/L or under. Risks rise by the degree of elevation, with the next highest risk range being 14–17, then 18–34, and above 35 indicating the highest risk for anything going wrong.

Serum iron and ferritin

Ferritin is to serum iron what files in a cabinet are to papers scattered on the desktop. Not exactly, but sort of. Ferritin is iron that has been put in storage. Serum iron is out and about and able to make mischief. Iron in the blood, in combination with vitamin B6, can create H_2S from the amino acid cysteine, also found abundantly in the blood.[126] Since GGT acts to break down glutathione and generate cysteine, seeing high GGT and high serum iron and/or ferritin is quite telling. It is a combination linked to a broad range of diseases.[127]

I think that each of the tests described above can give a unique window into potential sulfur metabolism issues. Because meaningful increases

123 Stephanie Seneff, et al. "Can glyphosate's disruption of the gut microbiome and induction of sulfate deficiency explain the epidemic in gout and associated diseases in the industrialized world?." *J Biol Phys Chem* 17.2 (2017): 53–76.

124 Duk-Hee Lee, Rune Blomhoff, and David R. Jacobs. "Review is serum gamma glutamyltransferase a marker of oxidative stress?." *Free Radical Research* 38.6 (2004): 535–539.

125 Ji-Seun Lim, et al. "Is serum γ-glutamyltransferase inversely associated with serum antioxidants as a marker of oxidative stress?." Free Radical Biology and Medicine 37.7 (2004): 1018–1023.

126 Jie Yang, et al. "Non-enzymatic hydrogen sulfide production from cysteine in blood is catalyzed by iron and vitamin B6." *Communications Biology* 2.1 (2019): 194.

127 Gerald Koenig and Stephanie Seneff. "Gamma-glutamyltransferase: a predictive biomarker of cellular antioxidant inadequacy and disease risk." *Disease Markers* (2015).

or decreases almost always fall within the lab reference range, the trick is to note the patterns *in combination with* the symptoms.

Lab Value	Optimal Range
Red blood cells (RBC)	Males: 4.5 to 5.5 (million cells/mm³) Females: 4.2 to 5.2
Hemoglobin	Males: 14 to 15g/dl Females: 13.5 to 14.5g/dl
Hematocrit	Males: 42 to 47% Females: 38 to 45%
Mean Corpuscular Volume (MCV)	82 to 94 cubic microns (fL)
Mean Corpuscular Hemoglobin (MCH)	28 to 30.9mcg
Gamma Glutamyl Transferase (GGT)	<14U/L
Homocysteine	7 to 8.5mmol/L
Vitamin B12	650 to >2000pg/mL
Ferritin	Males: 50 to 150ng;mL Females: 40 to 100ng/mL
Serum Iron	Males: 50 to 150mcg/dL Females: 40 to 140mcg/dL

Table 4. Useful Labs with Optimal Ranges

As you may have noticed, I don't use extensive lab testing to assess sulfur issues. Labs can help to confirm suspicions, but sulfur issues are predominantly identified and treated based upon clinical presentation, not lab results.

A final word about stool testing. I don't use it much. In naturopathic school I was taught a very straight-forward rule about running *any* lab test: If the result of the test is not going to change the treatment program, there is no need to run the test. If a patient has all the symptoms of a sulfur issue, I am going to implement the low-sulfur protocol *regardless* of any stool test results.

Stool testing: DNA tests vs culture tests

Many companies now offer DNA testing of stool to identify and quantify bacteria based upon the type and amount of bacterial DNA found in the stool. I recommend against this kind of testing.

DNA tests have two important limitations:

1. The test cannot distinguish between the DNA of living and dead organisms.

2. It is possible to count the wrong type of DNA as bacterial DNA.

If I do stool testing I will use stool culture tests. These are actually looking at the living organisms rather than simply their DNA. That way I know what is found is a living, viable, and potentially trouble-making bacteria, not just a DNA fragment passing through.

This doesn't mean that I never order stool tests. Not all gut issues are sulfur issues. If there is no response, or only minor response, to the low-sulfur protocol, then I may very well order stool testing to find out if there is some other overgrowth happening that needs to be addressed. My experience, though, is that addressing sulfur issues resolves most symptoms most of the time.

8

Additional Therapies

In this final chapter I'm going to run through some additional therapies I have patients employ during the low-sulfur protocol. A few of these are home therapies, and a few are therapies I'm using with patients in the clinic. I believe they are important, and for some people they elevate the benefits of the protocol to a whole new level. Many of the naturopathic physicians scattered around the country offer these same clinic-based therapies. It might take some homework to find the nearest option, but you might be able to find a clinic close to you that could support you with these more advanced therapies.

Home Therapies

Epsom Salt Baths

Most people, if they have considered Epsom salt baths at all, would think of them as either welcome relaxation or an inconvenience that isn't worth the effort. However, for people with sulfur metabolism issues, I consider these baths to be medicine.

Chemically, Epsom salt is magnesium sulfate. Magnesium is a great mineral for many reasons, as more than 300 reactions taking place in the body require the presence of magnesium. Evidence suggests that it lowers blood pressure,[128] reduces the risk of heart attacks,[129] reduces anxiety[130] and depression,[131] improves insomnia,[132] helps with regulation of blood sugar,[133] and much more. When you take the baths as I describe below, you will receive a healthy dose of magnesium in the process. But those are all fringe benefits of Epsom salt baths. For our purposes the key factor is not the magnesium, but the sulfate.

There has been one study on Epsom salt baths, and it was enough to convince me to make it a regular prescription for patients doing the low-sulfur protocol.[134] In that study, healthy adults had both their blood magnesium and sulfate levels measured before and after a nightly Epsom salt bath. The findings were interesting. Magnesium levels rose after the first few baths, and then leveled off. Sulfate levels, though, rose every night for an average of seven nights. After that, even with continued baths, sulfate levels stayed steady. This suggests there is a "pool" of sulfate in the blood that needs to be filled, and once filled it stays at a steady concentration even if more sulfate is available. These baths allow

---

128 Sun Ha Jee, et al. "The effect of magnesium supplementation on blood pressure: a meta-analysis of randomized clinical trials." *American Journal of Hypertension* 15.8 (2002): 691-696.

129 Fangzi Liao, Aaron R. Folsom, and Frederick L. Brancati. "Is low magnesium concentration a risk factor for coronary heart disease? The Atherosclerosis Risk in Communities (ARIC) Study." *American Heart Journal* 136.3 (1998): 480-490.

130 Neil Boyle, Clare Lawton, and Louise Dye. "The effects of magnesium supplementation on subjective anxiety and stress—a systematic review." *Nutrients* 9.5 (2017): 429.

131 N. Felice Jacka, et al. "Association between magnesium intake and depression and anxiety in community-dwelling adults: the Hordaland Health Study." *Australian and New Zealand Journal of Psychiatry* 43.1 (2009): 45-52.

132 David L. Watts. "The nutritional relationships of magnesium." *J Orthomol Med* 3.4 (1988): 197-201.

133 Giuseppe Paolisso, et al. "Magnesium and glucose homeostasis." *Diabetologia* 33.9 (1990): 511-514.

134 R.H. Waring. "Report on Absorption of magnesium sulfate (Epsom salts) across the skin." 2010. Epsom Salt Council Web site. http://www.epsomsaltcouncil.org/wp-content/uploads/2015/10/report_on_absorption_of_magnesium_sulfate.pdf. Accessed June 29, 2019.

both magnesium and sulfate to be absorbed through the skin so that they bypass the digestive tract.

Many dozens of patients and people around the world have emailed me to let me know that taking Epsom salt baths nightly for seven nights in a row has made an enormous difference to their digestion. The trick is that you have to use a lot of Epsom salt in each bath. *Four cups*, to be exact. That is the amount used in the study and is the amount I always recommend to my patients.

Why would baths improve digestion? I believe it is because Epsom salt baths supply the body with additional inorganic sulfate, which just needs to go through that PAPSS enzyme to become useful organic sulfate. Epsom salt baths supply sulfate while you are reducing dietary sulfur, but the beauty of them is that the sulfur they supply comes directly into the blood via skin absorption. The digestive tract is bypassed, and so are any bacteria that might want to make mischief out of that sulfur.

Coffee enemas

Few recommendations I make cause more looks of disgust—but there are also few where patients tell me oh-my-gosh how much better they feel after doing one. The first few times are always awkward and maybe messy and annoying. You can't judge the therapy as good or bad until you have done at least half a dozen, as that's how long it can take to get a routine down.

There is no end of ridicule of coffee enemas online. Beyond the obvious answer, which is to simply try them and see if you notice a benefit, another option is to go to the scientific literature and see if there is evidence for their benefit. Here is a brief review:

It is well established that coffee is high in a compound called chlorogenic acid.[135] This acid is a "bound" form of yet another compound called caffeic acid. Caffeic acid has lots of beneficial health effects, including

---

135 Margreet R. Olthof, Peter C.H. Hollman, and Martijn B. Katan. "Chlorogenic acid and caffeic acid are absorbed in humans." *The Journal of Nutrition* 131.1 (2001): 66-71.

the prevention of cancer,[136] promotion of collagen synthesis in skin for anti-aging effects,[137] reduction of inflammation,[138] and others.

When coffee meets up with the bacteria of the intestines, an enzyme called beta-glucuronidase splits the caffeic acid off of chlorogenic acid, allowing it to then be absorbed and create its various beneficial effects.[139] Caffeic acid is not the only beneficial component of coffee, and not the only benefit of the coffee enema.

Many are concerned that they will be amped up by the caffeine. My experience is that very few report this, and in fact most report that the enemas are relaxing. I recommend the first few be done in the morning in order to gauge reaction. It is not uncommon for people to then switch to doing them in the afternoon or evening. One study looked specifically at the amount of caffeine in the blood from drinking coffee vs doing a coffee enema with an equivalent amount of coffee, and it was found that the enema results in *3.5 times less* caffeine in the blood than drinking coffee.[140]

I have put the full instructions in Appendix A. While the process is quite simple, it occupies quite a bit of space when writing each step out. I will recommend them anywhere from a few times weekly to once daily depending on the severity of symptoms.

Earthing

This one is a newcomer on my list of recommendations, and I'm disappointed I didn't fully recognize its wide-ranging benefits earlier.

---

136 M.T. Huang and T. Ferraro. "Phenolic compounds in food and cancer prevention." *ACS Symposium Series* (USA). 1992.

137 C. Magnani, et al. "Caffeic acid: a review of its potential use in medications and cosmetics." *Analytical Methods* 6.10 (2014): 3203-3210.

138 Fernanda M. Da Cunha, et al. "Caffeic acid derivatives: in vitro and in vivo anti-inflammatory properties." *Free Radical Research* 38.11 (2004): 1241-1253.

139 M. Nardini, et al. "Absorption of phenolic acids in humans after coffee consumption." *Journal of Agricultural and Food Chemistry* 50.20 (2002): 5735-5741.

140 Supanimit Teekachunhatean, et al. "Pharmacokinetics of caffeine following a single administration of coffee enema versus oral coffee consumption in healthy male subjects." *ISRN Pharmacology* (2013).

The concept is very simple: spend at least 15 minutes each day—or longer if possible—with your bare feet touching the ground. Ideally this means touching grass or dirt, not just concrete. When we do this, negatively charged electrons flow from the earth, which has a few to spare, into our bodies. The health benefits have been thoroughly studied and documented. These benefits are extensive and include improved sleep, reduced pain and inflammation, lower stress, enhanced well-being, and others.[141] And on top of all that, keep in mind that a primary role of sulfate in the body is to provide negative charge that keeps water structured. Bringing in some additional negative charge in the form of electrons can't be a bad idea, and in fact maybe—*just maybe*—it accounts for some of the benefits associated with grounding.

Therapies in the Clinic

Ozone

Over half of my patients are utilizing ozone therapies in some form, usually intravenously, transdermally, or as an "ozone enema" in a technique called rectal insufflation. The health benefits of ozone are too extensive to go into fully here, but there are a few highly relevant specifics.

Ozone reacts with H_2S, producing water, SO_2, and oxygen.[142] Obviously water and oxygen are both fine things to have. The beauty of converting some of the H_2S to SO_2 is that the SO_2 can climb the ladder to SO_3 and then, via that SUOX enzyme, SO_4. So long as there is adequate molybdenum around for the SUOX enzyme to work properly, ozone shunts the symptomatic sulfur compound, H_2S, toward the much-needed SO_4.

---

141 Gaétan Chevalier, et al. "Earthing: health implications of reconnecting the human body to the earth's surface electrons." *Journal of Environmental and Public Health* (2012).

142 Sotirios Glavas and Sidney Toby. "Reaction between ozone and hydrogen sulfide." *The Journal of Physical Chemistry* 79.8 (1975): 779-782.

Pulsed Electromagnetic Field Therapy (PEMF)

The earth not only has a healthy supply of electrons to offer, but it also constantly generates a very low-level electromagnetic field (EMF). For the first few billion years, that field was the only field that mattered to life. By way of contrast, cell phones create an electromagnetic field that has a density over 2 *billion* times greater than that of the earth.[143] This doesn't take into account power lines, wi-fi, cell towers (with G5 being the most concerning of all), the "internet of things" like transmitting refrigerators, stoves, and even toasters, and a growing number of other EMF generators and transmitters. We exist in an ocean of these waves, and their cumulative impact on health is essentially unknown.

What *is* known is that exposure to EMFs can significantly alter stress hormone production,[144] and workers in power plants exposed to EMFs have an increased risk of depression, anxiety, stress, and poorer quality of sleep.[145] In fact, it has been proposed that the kinds of everyday EMFs we are all exposed to might be contributing directly to the disruption in the levels of healthy gut bacteria that fuels a great deal of this whole sulfur problem.[146]

Just as some chemicals act as toxins and other chemicals act as nutrients and medicines (remember that vitamins are chemicals, too), so too with EMFs. While many frequencies are harmful, other frequencies and intensities are beneficial to health. PEMF is a therapy that utilizes

143 Marko S. Markov, *Electromagnetic Fields in Biology and Medicine*. CRC Press, 2015.

144 S.M.J. Mortazavi, et al. "Occupational exposure of dentists to electromagnetic fields produced by magnetostrictive cavitrons alters the serum cortisol level." *Journal of Natural Science, Biology, and Medicine* 3.1 (2012): 60.

145 Majid Bagheri Hosseinabadi, et al. "The effect of chronic exposure to extremely low-frequency electromagnetic fields on sleep quality, stress, depression and anxiety." *Electromagnetic Biology and Medicine* 38.1 (2019): 96-101.

146 Marco Ruggiero and Stefano Aterini. "Electromagnetic fields." *Encyclopedia of Cancer* (2014): 1-5.

these beneficial frequencies to balance the autonomic nervous system.[147] This can reduce pain and stress, improve sleep, and generally enhance well-being. All of these are often indicated for individuals struggling with sulfur metabolism issues.

Alpha Stim

Alpha stim is delivered with a small, handheld electronic device. A small clip is attached to each earlobe, and the device sends a very low amperage electrical current of specific waveform and frequency in order to generate specific types of brain waves. Alpha waves are those associated with calm, relaxation, and focused attention. Alpha stim can be a helpful adjunct for those patients whose sulfur symptoms are predominantly anxiety, insomnia, or depression.[148] [149] All three are conditions for which alpha stim has received FDA approval as a treatment. Helping people out of these mental states can make it much easier to achieve lasting changes in digestive health, because mental states and digestion continuously feed back to each other to maintain either ongoing health or ongoing imbalances.

These supplemental therapies can be done along with the low-sulfur protocol to help the process, sometimes dramatically. But they are not essential, and many patients have had great results without doing any of these. Consider them enhancers. If I were going to prioritize them, I would say the home therapies are the most important, while the clinical

---

147 Emilio Baldi, Claudio Baldi, and Brian J. Lithgow. "A pilot investigation of the effect of extremely low frequency pulsed electromagnetic fields on humans' heart rate variability." *Bioelectromagnetics: Journal of the Bioelectromagnetics Society, The Society for Physical Regulation in Biology and Medicine, The European Bioelectromagnetics Association* 28.1 (2007): 64-68.

148 Timothy Culbert. "Perspectives on Technology-Assisted Relaxation Approaches to Support Mind-Body Skills Practice in Children and Teens: Clinical Experience and Commentary." *Children* 4.4 (2017): 20.

149 J.D. Feusner, S. Madsen, T.D. Moody, C. Bohon, E. Hembacher, S.Y. Bookeimer, and Bystritsky. "Effects of cranial electrotherapy stimulation on resting state brain activity." *Brain and Behavior.* 2012. Pp 1-10.

therapies are for the really tough-to-treat patients. Commit to seven nights of Epsom salt baths, then continue those a few nights a week thereafter. Try at least a few coffee enemas. And get your feet on the ground a little while each day. Then let the main food eliminations and supplement protocol do the rest of the work.

There you have it. You now know more about sulfur metabolism and how to treat its disruption than virtually every physician in the country. As the links between sulfur issues and various diseases become increasingly apparent, more doctors will, hopefully, be learning about it. Feel free to pass a copy of this book along to your family MD or ND. It could give them some new ideas about your care, and it just might help them help dozens of other patients as well.

Appendix A

Coffee Enema

The coffee should be prepared on a stovetop instead of in a coffee maker. It is imperative that you use organically grown coffee.

There are roasters that roast coffee specifically for use in coffee enemas—I know, odd, but thank goodness. The one our clinic uses is by http://sawilsons.com and there are others.

These can be done any time of the day, but I recommend the first one or two be done in the morning. The vast majority of people who do these do not get any caffeine stimulation from them, and, in fact, most find them relaxing. However, a few *do* get a caffeine buzz, so best to do the first few in the morning to gauge the response.

You should purchase a stainless steel enema bucket as well as silicon plastics that won't leech anything nasty when exposed to high temperature. Searching online with the words "stainless steel enema kit" will find several options. Assemble as the instructions say: attach the tubing to the bucket, thread the clamp onto the other end to about 5" from the end of the tube and *clamp it tight*. If you don't clamp it, then the coffee will just come running through the tube as soon as you pour it into the bucket.

With most kits there are a few different attachments that can fit onto the end of the tube where the coffee comes out. All you need to use is the short nozzle, which is typically about 3–4" and should look like this:

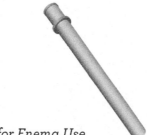

Figure 18. Nozzle for Enema Use

Add 2 tablespoons of the ground coffee to about 0.5L of filtered water in a pot. Bring that to a boil on the stove, then reduce to simmer, covered, for 15 minutes. Once it has brewed in this way, the coffee is ready. You don't really need a strainer. Just pour slowly into the enema bucket, allowing the coffee grounds to settle to the bottom of the pot as the liquid pours. If a few grounds pour in with the coffee it's no big deal.

Using an electric thermometer, bring the temperature down to 100°F-102°F. The thermometer gives a nearly instant temperature reading. Add ice cubes as needed to get the temperature right. In general, a single ice cube will drop the temperature by about 6°F in a standard enema bucket. You'll learn with time. Once at temperature, you are ready to go.

In the bathroom put a towel down for safety. You need a surface you can set the bucket on, so perhaps next to the sink or other shelf. Apply a small amount of lube to the enema tip. Coconut oil is a good option here, but any *all-natural and organic* lube or oil will work. It doesn't take much, just a light coat.

The next step is important. With the nozzle pointed into the sink, open the clamp so that coffee can fill the tube. Tip: With the nozzle in the sink and the clamp closed, lower the bucket below the level of the nozzle, *then* open the nozzle and raise the bucket up higher than the nozzle. This minimizes the amount of air that gets into the tube as the coffee flows through. As soon as it comes out the end and into the sink, close the clamp again. If you forget this step you'll be starting your enema with air, which is not a good thing.

Enema Extras

Once the coffee is at the correct temperature, there are a few things you can add to it to make the whole process even better for you.

1. Probiotic capsules—Purchase a refrigerated probiotic, preferably one that has both Lactobacillus and Bifidobacter. Open up 1 or 2 capsules and dump those into the coffee. It should be enough to total between 5 billion and 30 billion organisms.

2. Butyrate—There are a few supplements containing a salt of butyrate. I mentioned a few that I use in Chapter 6. Open up 2 capsules and add this to the coffee prior to use.

3. 3% Hydrogen peroxide—No more often than once weekly consider adding 1-3 tsp of preservative-free 3% hydrogen peroxide, purchased at a health food store. Start with 1 tsp the first time. The effect of it will be to slough off mucus from the lining of your bowel.

The next step is the one you've been waiting for. It's time to actually do the enema. There are a few options, and you'll need to find the one that works best for you. With the bucket now sitting on the sink counter or other surface about three feet off the floor and the base of the nozzle held with your dominant hand:

1. For those who are relatively agile, kneel down on one knee. Reach between your legs and gently insert the nozzle, advancing it slowly until it reaches the base of the nozzle. Next, being

mindful of the tubing, turn yourself around and simply lie down on your towel, making sure the nozzle stays inserted. You can now reach down and open up the clamp to let the coffee start to flow. Depending on the height of the bucket and the angle of the tubing, the coffee may or may not flow easily. Consider reaching up and holding the bucket above you, tipped very slightly in the direction of the outlet. You can raise and lower the bucket to regulate how fast the coffee flows.

2. For those who find it too clumsy to turn over and lie down with an enema tube inside, you can start by lying down on your back. From that position you will have to reach down and open the clamp. Again, consider reaching up and holding the enema bucket above you while it flows.

However you do it, I recommend you leave the nozzle inserted and the clamp open throughout the sessions.

Ideally the coffee is retained for 10–20 minutes before expelling it. This is not always easy. There will inevitably be waves of the urge for it to get out before then—it is actually great training for your nervous system to practice resisting that urge. Each wave can last from perhaps 10 seconds up to a minute or even longer. The waves tend to rise fairly gradually, stay for as long as they stay, then drop away gradually as well. During any given 15-minute retention enema there may be none at all, or there may be half a dozen.

When time is up or you just can't retain it any longer, reach down and close the clamp. If possible, I recommend ending your session between urges to expel, not during the urge. Next it is your choice: Remove the nozzle then stand up, or stand up then remove the nozzle. To minimize drips from the nozzle you should stand up first, remove the nozzle, immediately put it in the sink, and open the clamp to allow any residual coffee to drain out. Coil the tube in the sink basin as well. You can deal with the cleanup later.

You are now ready to sit down on the toilet for the expel. Don't be alarmed if it doesn't come out right away, or if obviously not all of it comes out initially. In fact, you should expect the coffee to come out, again, in waves. Allow about 10 minutes. Don't try to push the coffee out, just let it make its way out on its own.

When you feel the coffee is completely out, it is time to clean up. Disassemble all the parts. Use a concentrated soap such as Dr. Bronner's to wash the nozzle inside and out, and also wash the clamp. Next, with the tube coiled in the sink and detached from the bucket, pour some soap into one end of the tube. You can pinch the tube tightly with your fingers at that end, then slide your pinched fingers down the length of the tube to spread the soap end to end. Once that's done, run hot water into one end of the tube for about 30 seconds to allow it to flush all soap out of the tube completely.

The bucket is the last thing to clean. Squirt a decent amount of soap into the bucket and run hot water into it. Use your hand to wash up the sides of the bucket all the way around, then wash all around the bottom. Make sure every area is thoroughly washed. Pour the suds out, rinse with hot water, and put it all in storage until the next time.

Appendix B

Symptom Inventory

This inventory has two roles to play in this process. First, it should help to quantify just how closely your symptoms fit those I've seen correlate with sulfur metabolism issues. No one has all of these symptoms, and some might only have one or two. We're not trying to diagnose a sulfur problem based upon how many of the symptoms listed below you have. The goal here is to find out if any symptom you have is related to a sulfur issue.

The second point of this inventory is to make sure you have a record of your symptoms and how intense they are prior to starting the protocol. When you start introducing each food on the introduction list, you need to return to this list each time to make a note of the symptoms that did or didn't arise as a result. Many times I've had patients work through the protocol diligently only to end it with a splurge that exposes them to many sulfur sources at one time. Usually they report feeling quite miserable within a short time of that exposure, but they've lost the opportunity to learn which sulfur food or foods are the problem. The only way to find that out is with another two weeks of disciplined protocol.

There is a column for your symptoms before, then after the introduction of each of the 13 foods on the introduction list. Check the boxes of your symptoms before Day 1 of the protocol, then after each food introduction go through again and check any symptoms you notice on the day *of or after* each introduction.

	BEFORE	GARLIC	ONION	EGGS	KALE	BROCCOLI	CABBAGE	CAULIFLOWER	MEAT	ASPARAGUS	BRUSSEL SPROUTS	SPINACH	ALCOHOL	DAIRY
Night Sweats														
Hot Flashes														
Headaches														
Migraines														
Eczema														
Psoriasis														
Acne														
Dermatitis														
Rosacea														
Flushed face														
Anxiety														
Brain fog														
Panic attacks														
Constipation														
Diarrhea														
Reflux														
Bloating with meals														

	BEFORE	GARLIC	ONION	EGGS	KALE	BROCCOLI	CABBAGE	CAULIFLOWER	MEAT	ASPARAGUS	BRUSSEL SPROUTSS	SPINACH	ALCOHOL	DAIRY
Bloating on empty stomach														
Feeling of a bubble in digestion														
Generalized itching without visible rash														
Fatigue														
Chronic pain														
Fluid retention														
Low blood pressure														
Dizzy upon standing														
Slow heart rate														

Table 5. Symptom Review During Reintroductions

Author Bio

D r. Nigh is a 2001 graduate of the National University of Natural Medicine. He has a clinical focus on naturopathic oncology, Lyme disease, mold-related illness, SIBO, autoimmune illnesses, and of course the wide range of symptoms and conditions that are associated with impaired sulfur metabolism. In addition to his clinical work, he is a prolific writer and has spoken internationally on topics related to sulfur metabolism and its role in health and disease. His practice is at Immersion Health in Portland, Oregon, and can be found online at immersionhealthPDX.com

Comments, suggestions, and other feedback are welcome and encouraged. Submit them and get the latest news and updates at *DevilintheGarlic.com*.

Index

5-methyltetrahydrofolate-homo-
cysteine methyltransferase
reductase (MTRR), 14
basics of, 13
betaine-homocysteine-
N-methyltrans-ferase
(BHMT), 12–13
cystathionine beta synthase
(CBS), 16–17, 49–51, 100–101,
112
cystathionine gamma lyase
(CTH), 17, 51, 100–101, 112
homocysteine, 110–111
Hs3St1, 52
methylation genes and, 12–14
methylenetetrahydrofolate
reductase (MTHFR), 12–13, 51
polymorphisms in, 12–14,
16–18.47-53, 70, 96, 109
sulfation genes, 16–18
sulfite oxidase (SUOX). *see* separate entry
sulfur metabolism and, 47–53
glucosamine, 26, 52, 90
glucose, 95
glutathione
generation of hydrogen sulfide
and, 95–96
GGT enzyme and, 111
red blood cells and, 24
regulation of hydrogen sulfide,
45
sulfation pathway and, 14–15
supplementation, 51

glycine, 53, 56–57, 67–70
glycosaminoglycans (GAGs), 29
glyphosate
allowable concentrations of, in
US, 62–63
collagen and, 70–72
development of, 55–56
dysbiosis and, 64–67
glycine substitution and, 67–70
inflammatory bowel diseases
and, 79
iron and, 59
nutrient depletion and, 58–64
prevalence of, 57–58
pyrrole rings and, 72–73
structure of, 56–57
SUOX and, 70
gout, 41
gut bacteria
blood viscosity and, 77
glyphosate and, 64–65, 67
hydrogen sulfide and, 120–121
sulfite and, 19–22, 64–65, 67
sulfur-fixing bacteria and,
19–22, 64–65, 77, 99

H

heme, 42–43, 72
hemocrit, 107–108
hemoglobin, 72, 107–108, 109
heperan sulfate
connective tissue and, 26
heparanase and, 89
Hs3St1 gene and, 52

Made in the USA
Las Vegas, NV
08 November 2024

11375501R00095